Obstetrics and Gy Interview

Abbie Laing and Alexander Young

© 2015 MD+ Publishing

www.oginterview.com

Published by: MD+ Publishing

Cover Design: Alexander Logan

ISBN-10: 0993113842

ISBN-13: 978-0993113840

Printed in the United Kingdom

CONTENTS

Preface

Contributors

Chapter 1: The Basics

Chapter 2: Portfolio

Chapter 3: Clinical

Chapter 4: Communication

MORE ONLINE

www.oginterview.com

 Access Over 500 More Interview Questions

Head over to the Obstetrics and Gynaecology Interview website for the latest news on this year's interviews together with our online O&G interview questions bank featuring over 500 unique, interactive ST1 interview questions with comprehensive answers.

Created by high scoring, successful trainees the website and question bank can be accessed from your home computer, laptop or mobile device making your preparation as easy and convenient as possible.

Preface

ST1 run-through specialty training in obstetrics and gynaecology is a competitive process with around 600 applicants competing for just under 250 training posts each year. Competition ratios in the more popular deaneries such as London and Severn are in excess of 3:1 meaning that it is vitally important to understand both the application and interview process in order to achieve the highest ranking possible and secure your job preference.

Specialty interviews in medicine today are more similar to OSCEs than traditional job interviews with candidates required to rotate through a series of interview stations each testing components of the desirable criteria outlined in the national person specification.

Written by high-scoring candidates at previous obstetrics and gynaecology interviews this book has been specifically designed for doctors applying to obstetrics and gynaecology with a heavy focus on practice questions that are commonly asked at interviews.

Following a short introductory chapter covering an overview of the application process (we hope you already are aware of this!) and interview basics such as CV preparation and interview technique the remaining three chapters feature over 400 individual interview questions covering the structured portfolio, clinical and communication interview stations.

Improving your interview skills is best done through practice and this book can be used in pairs or groups to practise interview questions. If you prefer to prepare alone the clinical explanations, portfolio exercises and communication transcripts provide realistic insight into what is expected at ST1 obstetrics and gynaecology interviews.

For even more questions, an online question bank and plenty more resources remember to visit the companion website at:

www.oginterview.com

We hope this book helps boost your interview preparation.

Be confident and good luck.

Abbie and Alex

Contributors

Many thanks to the following obstetrics and gynaecology trainees who contributed to the text:

Imran Ahmed
Prisila Ahmed
Simi Bansal
Russell Biggs
Rachael Brooks
Jessica Cast
Andy Catton
Louise Channon
Daisy Clark
Charlie Crocker
Mark Davey
Jenny Davis
Claire Durrans
Annabelle Frost
Seuvandhi Gunasekera
Becks Hardcastle
Rosie Harrison
Naomi Harvey
Kirsten Herregods
Zara Jawad
Michelle Jie
Adeyinka Latunde-Dada
Sarah Law
Natalie Lee
Mridula Morje
Sadie Mullin
Jennie Naftel
Simrit Najjar
Hannah Oliver
Jessica Shepherd
Sarah Louise Smyth
Alice Strickland
Nazia Syed
Shehzad Syed
Laura Beth Welsh
Stephanie White
Gemma Williams

1 THE BASICS

THE BASICS

1.1 The ST1 Application Overview

Mid November - Early December	Application Window via ORIEL
December - January	Interview long listing takes place
Mid January - Mid February	All interviews take place
Mid March	All offers made
Late March	Deadline for holding offers
Mid April	Clearing

The ORIEL website recruitment portal

All applications for speciality training in Obstetrics and Gynaecology must be submitted through the online application forms via the ORIEL recruitment website (www.oriel.nhs.uk). Forms will not be accepted by post, e-mail or any other medium. This was designed for candidates to manage their application through a single portal and incorporates the following:

- An initial registration process, meaning applicants only need one log in for the entire recruitment year. Some parts of the completed registration will also get automatically transferred across to the obstetrics and gynaecology application to avoid repeating information.
- After registering, each applicant will have their own profile, it is through this that an applicant will complete the obstetrics and gynaecology application form and be informed if they are invited to interview or offered a training post.
- Booking interviews and assessment centres are managed through the portal.
- All available vacancies for speciality training are listed on the website.

The Application

Applicants will make a single application to their first preference deanery, with the opportunity to rank all other deaneries for consideration during the clearing process.

Once the application closes all candidates will have their eligibility assessed against criteria on the obstetrics and gynaecology person specification. Each deanery will use the same application form and all applicants that pass long listing will receive an interview.

Eligibility in the application is assessed against the obstetrics and gynaecology person specification.

The Obstetrics and Gynaecology Person Specification

While the format and location of how applicants are selected into obstetrics and gynaecology specialty training has drastically changed over the last ten years the underlying characteristics and desirable criteria for selection has not. The Person Specification outlines the requirements necessary for entry into obstetrics and gynaecology specialty training and has not changed significantly over the last ten years. The Person Specification is divided into two parts: Entry Criteria and Selection Criteria.

The entry criteria lists what is required to be eligible to apply for obs and gynae and this includes possessing a medical degree, having (or expecting to have) obtained your foundation training competencies, being in good health and being able to fluently speak english.

The selection criteria is the more important section as it is against this that applicants will be scored during the application and interview process. The selection criteria lists both 'essential' and 'desirable' criteria in certain domains together with the stage of the selection process these will be assessed and what evidence is required to score points. There are six key domains against which applicants will be scored and it is important to be aware of these together with the 'desirable' criteria for each to know how to score maximum points during the selection process and what evidence may be required.

- Qualifications
- Clinical Skills
- Academic Skills
- Personal Skills
- Probity – professional integrity
- Commitment to specialty – learning and personal development

Application Structure

After registering through ORIEL candidates will be able to add information to the application system when it opens mid-November to early December each year.

The Oriel application consists of 11 sections for obstetrics and gynaecology. Each section is marked against the person specification and it is very important that you compare your answers to this. Section 7 (Evidence) and section 8 (Supporting) are the most important sections to answer well and in sufficient detail. An overview of each section can be found on the next page.

The ORIEL Application Structure

11 sections need to be completed in full prior to submitting your application.

1	Personal	Contact information and personal details
2	Eligibility	Professional Registration, language skills, right to work in the UK
3	Fitness	Criminal Records and Fitness to Practice
4	References	Three references who have supervised your training during the last 2 years. One referee must be a current or most recent consultant or educational supervisor
5	Competencies	Achievement of foundation competence Evidence of primary medical qualification: MBBS or equivalent Evidence of Advanced Life Support Certificate from the Resuscitation Council UK or equivalent
6	Employment	Full employment history UK/ Overseas Any gaps in employment of longer than 4 weeks within 3 years preceding the start date of the post, must be accounted for
7	Evidence	Additional undergraduate degrees and qualifications Post-graduate degrees and qualifications Additional achievements, prizes awards and distinctions Training courses attended Career Progression. Evidence to show career progression is consistent with personal circumstances. 18 months or less experience in O&G (excluding foundation modules) is required for ST1 application.
8	Supporting	Clinical knowledge and expertise Research, teaching and quality improvement Presentations and publications Management and information technology Commitment to speciality Learning and personal development Achievements relevant to a career in O&G Other achievements and personal skills
9	Preferences	Application directly to one deanery
10	Equality	Equality and diversity monitoring form
11	Declaration	Declarations and submission

Section 7: Evidence

The evidence section on the application form includes 5 areas. The first four will make up most of your score for this section. The higher your score the better your application.

Additional undergraduate degrees and qualifications	Intercalated BSc /Equivalent Other degrees BSc /BA Includes Grade
Postgraduate degrees and qualifications	Other degrees /diplomas A PhD or MD should only be listed in this section that has been awarded for defending a thesis
Additional achievements, prizes, awards and distinctions	Include specialty and qualifying distinction Indicate if awarded as an undergraduate or a postgraduate
Training courses attended	Include relevant training courses to O&G Include courses currently being undertaken ALS
Career progression	The maximum experience in Obstetrics and Gynaecology for application at ST1 level is 18 months in any country. This does not include experience in foundation modules.

Section 7 scoring systems
When the application is independently scored marks are awarded based on a set scoring system. If you are aware of the requirements well ahead of time you can spread your achievements across each of the scoring domains in order to score as many high marks as possible.

A few example scoring systems for the evidence section of the application are shown on the next page.

> ᗝᗝ **Prepare Early and Be Honest**
>
> Remember to prepare your application well ahead of time. While scoring maximum marks in one area is good it is important that you score highly in each section to ensure a high overall application score. Whatever achievements you list in the sections 7 or 8 make sure you have evidence to support them as any fraudulent answers may be reported to the GMC.

Postgraduate degrees and qualifications example scoring

Degree /Qualification	Rank	Example scoring system
PhD or DPhil Doctor of Philosophy	Highest score	10
MD Doctor of Medicine - two year original research-based	Middle/High score	8
MPhil Master of Philosophy	Middle score	6
Single year post-graduate course (eg MSc, MA, MRes)	Middle score	5
MD Doctor of Medicine - dissertation	Lower Score	4
Post-graduate diploma (This does not include MRCP)	Lower score	3

Additional achievements example scoring

Additional achievements, prizes, awards and distinctions	Rank	Example scoring system
Awarded national prize related to medicine	Highest score	10
High achievement award for primary medical qualification (eg honours or distinction)	Middle/High score	8
More than one prize / distinction / merit related to medical course	Middle score	6
One prize / distinction / merit related to parts of medical course	Middle score	4
Scholarship / bursary / equivalent awarded during medical course	Lower Score	2

Section 8: Supporting Evidence

The supporting evidence section of the application form encompasses other areas relevant to the person specification for obstetrics and gynaecology. This part of the application can typically ask for short answers in prose. Section 8 is divided into 8 distinct areas closely following those of the person specification.

Clinical knowledge and experience	Details of your level of experience Level of competence Training priorities
Research, teaching and quality improvement	Audits Q:I projects Teaching
Presentations and publications	Presentations at regional or national level Presentations at local level Publications in journals Other publications
Management and information technology	Descriptive experiences of managerial roles or working in a team Experience with information technology
Commitment to speciality	Evidence of commitment Career objectives
Learning and personal development	Setting realistic goals Demonstrating commitment
Achievements relevant to a career in O&G	Examples outside of medicine of team working, problem solving or hobbies that might improve surgical skills like textile work
Other achievements and personal skills	Achievements outside of medicine

Section 8 scoring systems

As with section 7 your answers will be scored against a set marking criteria based on the perceived level of your achievements. On the next page you will find some example scoring systems for section 8.

 More Online

A full lists of the scoring systems for each section can be found on the *OG Interview* website (www.oginterview.com). You can also find lots of free resources to help you gain maximum marks.

THE BASICS

Clinical audit and quality improvement example scoring

Clinical Audit / Quality Improvement	Rank	Example scoring system
Designed led and implemented change through a completed audit and QI project and presented the completed results at a meeting	Highest score	10
Designed led and implemented change through a completed audit and QI project; but without presenting the results	Middle/High score	8
Actively participated in a completed audit or QI project and presented results at a meeting	Middle score	6
Actively participated in a completed audit or QI project: but without presenting the results	Middle score	4
Participated only in certain stages of an audit or QI project	Lower Score	2

Poster and presentation example scoring

Degree /Qualification	Rank	Example scoring system
Oral presentation at a national or international medical meeting	Highest score	6
Shown more than one poster at a national or international medical meeting	Highest score	6
Oral presentation at a regional medical meeting	Middle score	4
Shown one poster at a national or international medical meeting	Middle score	4
Shown one or more posters at a regional medical meeting	Lower Score	2
Given an oral presentation or shown one or more posters at a local medical meeting	Lower score	2

THE BASICS

THE BASICS

ST1 O&G APPLICATION TOP TIPS

✚ Some questions are mandatory.

✚ Some sections have a strict word limit.

✚ All parts of the application are needed to be completed prior to submission.

✚ Completion of MRCOG Part 1 is not a mandatory requirement for ST1 application.

1.2 | The ST1 Interview Overview

The Obstetrics and Gynaecology interview consists of three stations each lasting 15 minutes. Like the application, each station is designed to assess the selection criteria of the person specification. There are typically two to three examiners per station.

The stations for the ST1 Obstetrics and Gynaecology Interview are:

- **Structured Interview (*Portfolio*) Station**
- **Clinical Skills Station**
- **Communication Skills Station**

Each interview station is scored out of 40 based on both the content of your answers and the way in which you deliver them (communication skills). The minimum mark to be appointable is 60 and your application score also contributes to your final overall score and subsequent ranking.

For the clinical skills and communication skills stations you will be required to read a laminated scenario before entering the examination room. The time you take to read this scenario is included in your interview time.

ᐸᐳ Key Interview Information

- 3 stations, 15 minutes per station
- Each station is marked out of 40
- A minimum score of 60 is required to be considered appointable

---

THE BASICS

Structured interview station

At the structured interview station two examiners will ask you questions about different parts of your portfolio. The reason this is called a structured interview station is because each candidate is asked the same questions based around their portfolio. Questions will typically follow areas of the person specification such as 'teaching', 'audit', 'leadership' etc.

 10 Common Structured Interview Station Questions

These are the most common questions asked at O&G interview stations. Make sure you learn these well. Chapter 2 of this book covers the structured interview and features answers to all these questions:

1. Define Audit
2. Tell me about an audit that you have undertaken, take me through the steps.
3. Tell me about your teaching experience
4. What do you understand about changes being made to the Consultant job in O&G?
5. What do you understand about the training MATRIX?
6. Tell me what is expected from you as an ST1 level in O&G according to the MATRIX
7. Tell me about a piece of research you have undertaken
8. Take me through your portfolio
9. Do you think it will be a good thing for Consultants to be covering LW as well as senior registrars?
10. How have you demonstrated your commitment to O&G?

STRUCTURED INTERVIEW STATION TOP TIPS

➕ It is very important that your portfolio folder is organised logically and clearly. Use a clear contents page at the front that outlines the topics in order. The examiners may only have 5 minutes to read your portfolio so it is important for it to be user friendly.

➕ You may also be required to direct them to specific sections when answering questions, for example they may want to see evidence of a recent audit. You will need to be able to show them exactly where this is in your portfolio.

Clinical skills station

In the clinical skills scenario you will typically be asked to review a patient and make a clinical plan. You will need to act as though this is real life and you are not being watched. Usually you will need to use a structured '**ABCDE**' approach, take a history and examine the patient. The examiners will then ask you clinical questions at the end. The clinical scenario is designed to assess knowledge at the level of an F2 and will not be based on a detailed obstetric or gynaecological case.

Questions will test your clinical judgement under pressure (another area of the person specification) and interviewers may well ask you quick-fire questions and push the best candidates to really test their knowledge.
Interviewers simply want to know that you are safe and are able to safely and succinctly assess and identify emergent and life-threatening conditions that might affect obstetric and gynaecological patients.

CLINICAL STATION TOP TIPS

 The questions in the clinical chapter of this book cover most of the main emergent scenarios. Use an ABCDE approach to structure your answer and remember to call for senior help if required.

Communication scenario

In the communication station you will typically be asked to speak to a patient or relative who has a concern. An actor will play the part of the patient or relative and you will need to communicate with them effectively. The examiners do not typically speak to you in this scenario but rather assess the interaction in silence.

The communication chapter of this book features realistic transcripts of some of the commonly asked communication scenarios. Integrated into these transcripts are some key knowledge topics and explanations.

COMMUNICATION STATION TOP TIPS

 Use open questions to begin the consultation, gathering key information and ensure you know the patient's ideas, concerns and expectations before delivering any information in simplistic and empathetic terms.

1.3 | CV and Portfolio

Up until now you may have kept a fairly arbitrary CV and portfolio chronicling all of the courses you have attended and past glories as a school prefect. You probably have a vast amount of information and knowing how to present this in a manner that is both engaging and easy for interviewers to read can be tricky.

In this section we will give you the tools to help you write and layout your CV and structure your portfolio in a way that will maximise the impression you leave on interviewers and, hopefully, points scored at the structured interview portfolio station. We recommend structuring your CV and portfolio in an identical order to avoid interviewer confusion. We therefore consider both the CV and portfolio together in the below sections.

1.3.1 | Layout

Knowing how to present your achievements so that interviewers spot them quickly and award you points is an art. A regular CV is usually two to three pages in length covering your previous employment, skills and extracurricular achievements. For medics a CV can go beyond ten pages in order to match the person specification and demonstrate achievements in all the domains necessary to be deemed an appointable candidate. The below layout is based on the authors' collective knowledge having read and reviewed over one thousand medical CVs and reviewed portfolios at interview courses.

Structure and Headings

The first step is deciding upon what headings you are going to use for your CV and portfolio. For ST1 obstetrics and gynaecology we recommend sticking closely to the themes described in the Person Specification to help interviewers to quickly see what you have demonstrated in each of these domains. We recommend the below headings as a good starting point:

- Personal Details
- Qualifications
- Achievements
- Appointments/Jobs
- Publications
- Presentations
- Teaching
- Management
- Research
- Audits
- Logbook
- Courses
- Extracurricular
- Statement of Intent
- References

CV Front Page

This might sound obvious but the front page is the first thing that the interviewers will see when they pick up your CV. It's kind of a big deal. There are two real options for your front page: a cover page or straight into the first page.

Both options have advantages and disadvantages. A cover page looks neat and should feature your full name followed by qualifications to draw attention to your academic achievements. Going straight to your first page has the advantage of focussing more attention on it and reducing the amount of pages the interviewer needs to flick through. There is no right or wrong answer, just personal preference.

Cover page aside the first page should be composed of your personal details and qualifications taking up half the page. The remainder of the page should demonstrate your biggest achievements and key selling points.

The first page should be treated as the front page of a newspaper showing your most important headlines so that interviewers can immediately see what you are offering before they start looking a individual sections. This not only saves time but also gives a great first impression which is likely to stick in the interviewer's mind as he/she looks through the rest of your CV.

Ordering Your CV and Portfolio

Though your CV and portfolio should cover the domains outlined in the Person Specification (as this is what you will be scored against) there is no necessity to follow any set order for presenting these in your CV or portfolio.

We recommend putting your best areas towards the front. Interviewers have limited time to review your CV/Portfolio and will have looked through lots of others on the day. Putting your best bits first ensures that they are not skimmed through or overlooked by a tired/bored interviewer.

In practical terms if your 'teaching' section is much stronger than your 'audit' section then put 'teaching' ahead of 'audit',

Subheadings

The majority of 'main' headings can be easily divided into subheadings that make life even easier for interviewers.

For example 'presentations' can be quickly divided into 'Posters' and 'Podium' and the again into 'International', 'National', 'Regional' and 'Local'.

Chronology

When adding content under the above heading put the most recent events and work at the top with other points descending in date. This shows your most recent work easily and is the accepted format in most CVs.

THE BASICS

1.3.2 | Content

Once you are happy with your layout it is time to start adding in all of your work and achievements.

Certifications First

When arranging your portfolio make sure you put your medical degree, GMC and other key certifcates at the front mirroring the 'qualifications' section of your CV.

First Page Headlines

As suggested put your best achievements on the front page under a generic heading such as 'achievements' or 'positions of responsibility', highlight your role and give a brief description (a single line) of what this entailed. These achievements can be subsequently duplicated within their corresponding section (e.g. publication, presentation etc) and provide a quick way for interviewers to immediately see your key selling points.

 Key Achievements

Book Reviewer: For Hodder-Arnold and Oxford University Press
Rota Organiser: O&G F2 and SHO Royal Hospital 2014-15
Volunteer: RCOG School Career's Day
School Prefect: Hogwarts' School

Summary Sheets

Rather than printing out every single work-based assessment create a summary table giving an overview of the number of WBAs that you have achieved. You may also wish to include quotes from some of your 360 feedback that might help to back up your answers to questions such as 'what do your colleagues think about your communication skills?'.

How Do I Give Evidence of Audit?

Whereas publications, presentations and course attendance often come with hard copy certificates it is unlikely you will have anything official to prove that you completed an audit or quality improvement project. If this is the case use an audit summary (see box) and also print off the slides from any presentations you might have given at local departmental audit meetings.
Summaries can also be employed for research, WBAs and operations. You just need to create and print off the summary sheet and put it in the corresponding section of your portfolio.

> ✏️ **Using an Audit Summary**
>
> **Completed Audit Cycles:**
> *Title:* Enhanced Recovery Programme for Post-Op Patients
> *Location:* My Royal Hospital August 2012
> *Role*: Audit lead and identified the problem
> *Criteria:* Gynae ERP meets local guidelines
> *Implementing change:* Education and implementation of proforma
> *Outcome:* Average inpatient stay reduced from 5.4 to 3.5 days post op. Reducing bed costs (£225/day). Currently doing re-audit looking at patient satisfaction scores.

Should I Include…?

If this is your second, third or fourth attempt at the interviews you may well have amassed a significant volume of historic audits that you may well have forgotten about.

Keeping these in your CV/Portfolio is ok but remember that you will need to be able to discuss them in detail if you are asked about them. Removing audits from over 24 months ago is also ok but make sure you are prepared to talk about what you did in this time if you are asked.

Indeed, even if this is your first sitting including your 10M swimming certificate and Duke of Edinburgh bronze award is unlikely to score you any points but will certainly take up space. Be ruthless and try to cut our anything that won't score you points.

Verbosity

Try not to put in too much text. This takes up space and it is unlikely to be read in its entirety by interviewers with limited time. Try to explain any things such as teaching events with focused bullet points outlining what you did and what you gained.

1.3.3 | Design

Finally once you are happy with both your layout and content it is time to present your CV and portfolio in a way that will make the interviewers' life as easy as possible to find key information.

Font

Size 18 Comic Sans is not going to give a good impression. Arial is simple and sized at 10 or 11 will give you a good economy of words per page. Other options are Helvetica or Times New Roman. Again there is no right or wrong option (other than comic sans) so try a few different variations to see which suits you best. Whatever you choose stick to this font for the entire CV and don't mix and match.

Colours

Colours are not required but can help draw attention to areas of your CV. In a similar vein to 'Font' try to keep things simple and, if you are going to use a colour, try to stick to one only and use it to help divide sections or to offset the header/footer area.

Dividers

A simple line can help to split up sections and divide your CV preventing it from becoming a giant block of text. Again there are a few options involving colours or boxes so try a few and decide which you like, but remember, keep it simple. Within your portfolio numbered or coloured split dividers should be used to break up sections and make it easy for interviewers to quickly flick to different sections.

Headers/Footers

The header/footer area should feature your name on each page (in case the interviewers forget). Don't go overboard and grey scaling the text can prevent it from drawing attention away from your content.

Highlight Your Name

For publications, presentations or any section where there are multiple authors make sure you highlight your name in bold text to make it stand out allowing interviewers to quickly spot your role.

Review, Edit, Review

Once you are near happy review your CV and portfolio and check for spelling errors. Get someone else to do the same and edit it again after a short break. Try to get your CV and portfolio sorted by Christmas so that you can concentrate on practising your interview technique.

Being 'good' at interviews is a skill and as with all skills it will get better with understanding how to improve and then practising. Studies have shown that impressing interviewers and scoring highly at interviews is as much about how you communicate and convey your answer as much as it is about the content of the answer itself.

1.3.4 Example CV Layout and Headings

PERSONAL DETAILS

Date Of Birth:

Address:
Telephone:
Email:
GMC Registration:

EDUCATION & QUALIFICATIONS

Postgraduate Qualifications

Medical Qualification

School Qualifications

ACHIEVEMENTS/POSITIONS OF RESPONSIBILITY

PRIZES/AWARD

END OF PAGE 1

APPOINTMENTS

Foundation Year 1

Foundation Year 2

AWARDS, SCHOLARSHIPS & PRIZES

PRESENTATIONS

International

National

Regional

Local

PUBLICATIONS

Peer-Reviewed

Abstracts

THE BASICS

Books and Book Chapters

Non peer-reviewed

TEACHING

Postgraduate Degrees

Courses

National

Local

MANAGEMENT

AUDITS AND RESEARCH

COURSES ATTENDED

Certifications

Other Courses

MEMBERSHIPS

ELECTIVE & VACATION PLACEMENTS

EXTRACURRICULAR ACHIEVEMENTS

LOGBOOK SUMMARY

CAREER AIMS

REFERENCES

 More Online: www.oginterview.com

- A downloadable CV template can be found on the website
- Even more articles covering CV and portfolio preparation are regularly added to the blog and newsletter

1.4 | Interview Technique

Making an impression and scoring highly at the interview stations is as much about your overall interview technique as it is about the content of your answers. Coming across as confident and a 'good' candidate is a skill and can be improved with practise. Try to utilise the below interview techniques when practising your answers.

1.4.1 | Interview Communication Skills

Interviews are not just about facts and it is important that you are aware of other factors that will contribute to your interview score and the overall impression that you leave the interviewers with.

Body language (Non-Verbal Communication Skills)

Body language is extremely important and plays a pivotal role in effective communication. It can be difficult to know how to sit, who to look at or what to do with your arms during an interview.

Sitting
A number of studies have identified the position of sitting slightly forward feet planted on the ground with hands crossed or fingers locked and forearms resting on your thighs as being the optimum position for interviews. This position makes you look calm and ready and is in between leaning over the table and slouching back in your chair. This position can be maintained for the majority of the interview and allows you to sit back slightly between questions or at the end of the interview.

Smile
Smiling has been shown to increase attractiveness by a factor of ten and will also convey confidence and personality to the interviewers. While you may be extremely nervous make sure you smile when you greet the panel and try to show enthusiasm when talking about why you want to study medicine or something that you are passionate about.

Eye Contact
Ensure that you make eye contact with the interviewers from the start. If you find holding eye contact difficult practice focussing on peoples' eyebrows when you talk to them (the eye of the other person cannot discriminate whether you are looking at their eye or eyebrow due to proximity). When listening to questions concentrate on the interviewer asking the questions, nodding to show understanding. When giving your answers make sure you make eye contact with all the panel and not just the interviewer asking the question. At least one of the interviewers will be making notes or scoring you so do not be phased if they do not maintain eye contact.

Hands
From the initial handshake to using hand gestures to enforce points your hands can help to demonstrate confidence and conviction if used correctly. Upon entering the room respond to handshakes if offered and look the interviewers in the eyes. Keep your hands on your knees or lap when listening to questions and raise them when making a firm point.

Appearance
For male applicants: smart shoes, smart suit, plain shirt and plain tie. For women a smart skirt or trousers and a shirt with or without a suit jacket will be fine. It is important that you appear smart and dress as a registrar would when seeing patients in a clinic.

Active Listening
When being asked questions sit attentively. Movements such as tilting your head or nodding in understanding demonstrate active listening and will make you appear more engaging to the interviewers.

Verbal Communication Skills
Once you have mastered body language it is time to analyse how you deliver your responses to the interviewers. An excellent answer delivered in a quiet, stuttering manner will score less than one given with gusto.

Vocal Clarity
Project your voice beyond the interviewers, sit upright and speak clearly. You will be nervous initially and may hear your voice waiver. This is entirely normal and you will settle in to things after you begin speaking.

Length of Response
Stopping yourself from talking when nervous can be extremely difficult, however, interviewers are likely to lose concentration after around 3 minutes of listening to you talk. Most structured points can be given within 2-3 minutes leaving time for further questions.

Speed
Some people talk quickly others talk slowly. Try to find a balance and don't be afraid to pause to consider the question before jumping into your answer.

Vocal Tonality
Changing your inflection and emphasising words prevents interviewers from getting bored. Think about how quickly you lose interest when speaking to someone talking about something in a monotonous, single tone voice and then think about someone who changes their tone and emphasises words. Less easy to fall asleep, right?

Enthusiasm
Following on from tonality and word emphasis make sure that you are enthusiastic when delivering your answers. Smiling and tonality make up a large portion of this and the rest is about overcoming nerves and remembering that you

should be excited about obs and gynae and the things that you have done.

Positive Answers

When answering structured, portfolio questions be sure to turn everything into a positive even when asked about weaknesses or receiving criticism. Similarly try to avoid using phrases like 'I think' or 'Maybe I would' when asked about your management in the clinical station. Be positive and use confident phrases such as 'I would manage this patient by...'. Take a look at the list of action words at the end of this chapter for more examples of how to verbally demonstrate confidence.

 Vocal Tonality Practice

The sentence 'I want to be a gynaecologist' can be interpreted in a number of ways depending on the tonality of the delivery. For instance a person increasing their inflection towards the end of the sentence suggests a question: 'I want to be a gynaecologist?'. While delivery with a firm tone suggests more of a statement: 'I want to be a gynaecologist!'. More over emphasis of words can dramatically alter the sentence structure; 'I WANT to be a gynaecologist', 'I want to BE A GYNAECO-LOGIST'.

TOP TIPS

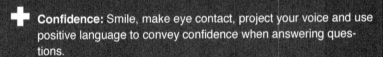 **Confidence:** Smile, make eye contact, project your voice and use positive language to convey confidence when answering questions.

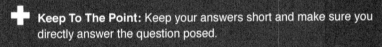 **Keep To The Point:** Keep your answers short and make sure you directly answer the question posed.

THE BASICS

THE BASICS

1.4.2 | Interview Frameworks

Although you cannot predict and prepare for every question that might be asked at interview it is helpful to have a framework to answer specific portfolio-type questions. Roughly speaking questions asked at any type of interview can be categorised into motivational, situational, opinion and specific. Having a framework will help you to logically structure your answers for both basic and more challenging questions and help you think under pressure.

Different question types will require different frameworks. Question types fall into categories or domains based on what the interviewers are testing. Whichever framework you use you should be able to cut your answer down to 3-4 solid, personal experiences and reflect on each. Remember these frameworks are guides only and it is fine to use a different way to structure your answer or only use part of the framework. You can find examples of these frameworks in action in the structured interview (portfolio) chapter.

Motivational and Experiential: CAMP

e.g. Why O&G? Tell me About Your Work Experience

Clinical
Academic
Management
Personal

Problem-Solving Questions: SPIES

e.g. How would you deal with this problem?

Situation
Problem
Initiative
Escalate
Support

Situational and Skills Questions: STAR

e.g. How have you shown leadership? Have you been part of a team?

Situation
Task
Action
Result

1.4.3 | Interview Circuit Technique

It is important to remember that you will be rotating around an interview circuit with other candidates behind and ahead of you. Your starting station will be random and there is no 'good' or 'bad' first station. If you think an interview station has not gone as well as you had hoped don't dwell on it as you will be going directly into a new station afterwards. Below are some further tips specific for the OSCE-style of interview.

Don't Forget to...

Read The Question: Ensure you read or listen to each question and understand what the interviewers want from your answer.

Time Management: Make sure your answers are succinct and focussed. Time is limited as you will be moving stations and there will be little time to waffle on.

Don't Panic: If a station goes badly forget about it and give the next station your best shot.

Actors: Try to treat the actors seriously and listen and respond to them. You will be assessed on your empathy and communication skills so ensure you employ the active listening suggestions listed above in the communication skills section and use phrases such as 'I understand', 'I am sure that must be difficult for you', 'I am sorry to hear that' to directly demonstrate empathy and understanding.

Content of Answers

Regardless of the interview type, interviewers will want to know about your experience, your extracurricular activities, how you deal with pressure, how you resolve problems and whether you can demonstrate empathy.

Be Personal and Specific: Talking about generic things like 'I saw a patient having blood taken' or 'I have leadership skills' will not score you as many points as using personal experiences and reflecting on what you learned.

Structure Your Answers: Structuring your answers into 3-4 headlines will make it easy for interviewers to follow and prevent you from wasting time with waffle.

Common Questions: Write out example answers for common questions and then practise them. Try not to be too scripted rather work on your delivery and enthusiasm once you are happy with your content.

Use Your CV As A Guide: Interviewers may ≠have missed key parts of your CV or portfolio. Make sure that you talk about all the best points that you have written down and do not assume that the interviewers have read it. Your CV should be structured to say why you want to do obs and gynae, what work experience you have done and what you know about O&G training; these are also three of the most commonly asked questions!

THE BASICS

Show Your Working: For tough ethical or decision-making questions be sure to talk through what you are thinking. There is often no right or wrong answer rather the interviewers want to see you logically discussing both sides of the argument or problem.

Be Positive and Sell, Sell, Sell: Interviewers want to hear how great you are and it is important that you are not bashful or reserved when telling them about your achievements and why they should choose you. Turn everything into a positive and don't undersell yourself.

Don't Give An Overview: Outlining how you are going to answer a question or explaining your framework is unnecessary and risky. One particularly awkward moment occurred when an interview candidate confidently stated there were three reasons he wanted to be a gynaecologist only for him to be unable to recall the third!

Read The Instructions: The communication and clinical stations will provide you with written information upon entering the station. Remain calm and read the instructions or scenario carefully. Try to mentally highlight the important points and understand what they want you to do.

Answer The Question: This might seem silly but it is amazing how often candidates do not give a direct answer or go off-topic. Make sure you understand what has been asked and avoid giving a long-winded introduction.

Other Factors

The thought of the interview can be scary and there are some other variables that you will need to consider such as how you are going to get to the venue and what happens when you get there. You will be sent detailed information regarding the interview process and venue in good time. Below are some top tips for how to stay calm around the time of the interview itself.

The Night Before: You may have chosen to stay in the city before your interview or you may be travelling up on the day. Whatever you have chosen to do ensure that you have your clothes prepared, shoes shined and know where and when you need to be at the interview location. Ensure you have all the required documentation and identification required well ahead of time. Relax and get a good night's sleep the evening before, making sure you set your alarm to wake up in good time the next morning.

On the Day: Get up in good time and have a proper breakfast. Make sure you factor in traffic if you are driving to the interview location. Upon arriving at the venue you will need to register so that the organisers know that you have arrived. Occasionally your interview time slot may have been altered. If this is the case don't panic and go with the flow. There will be refreshments provided and you will be told where you can wait before the interview.
An interviewer or facilitator will usually call you in once they are ready. Upon entering greet and shake hands with the interviewers ensuring that you try to appear as confident as possible.

1.4.4 | What The Interviewers Say

We asked a selection of experienced interviewers to give their opinions on what makes the difference between a good candidate and an excellent candidate. Here is what they had to say:

> "The biggest challenge of any interview candidate is answering the questions posed in a way that incorporates your best points in a concise format. Your interview station time is limited. This can be especially difficult when asked a very broad, open question such as 'Why should we choose you?'"

> "As an interviewer I can tell you that the best candidates are the ones who answer the questions posed in a logical and structured format and who have clearly thought about how they will answer the common questions."

> "Candidates who appear confident, with good body language and vocal intonation have often acquired this through previous interview or public speaking experiences. The more formal interview practice that you do the more relaxed you will be on the day of the real thing and this will translate into a more confident performance."

> "Ask any interviewer what separates the best and worst interview candidates and they are likely to respond with a single word 'waffle'. (Most) interviewers are human and will be interviewing candidates for the entire day of interviews. Think about the last time you spoke with someone, maybe a friend or relative, who told a long and boring story. It can be difficult to stay focused and retain information when candidates talk for longer than 3-4 minutes or repeat themselves. Preparing and practising questions with a set framework will help you to get across your best selling points in a concise format."

> "Some candidates struggle to sell themselves and feel awkward or boastful when asked why they would be a good doctor or why they should be chosen. The best way around this is to bring objectivity into the answer. For example, rather than saying 'I am a great leader' you may be more comfortable saying 'feedback from my supervisors and peers highlights my strong leadership skills'. You should of course back this up with a specific example such as when you captained a sports team or led a crash call."

THE BASICS

1.4.5 CV and Interview Action Words

One way to really sell yourself in both your application and interview is to make sure you choose appropriate action words that match the corresponding skills that are being assessed.

Below is a list of action words that you may wish to use when writing your application and CV and when answering interview questions to make your answers sound more positive and assertive.

Leadership Skills

Administered
Appointed
Approved
Assigned
Attained
Authorized
Chaired
Considered
Consolidated
Contracted
Controlled
Converted
Coordinated
Decided
Delegated
Developed
Directed
Eliminated
Emphasized
Enforced
Enhanced
Established
Executed
Generated
Handled
Headed
Hired
Hosted
Improved
Incorporated
Increased
Initiated
Inspected
Instituted
Led
Merged
Motivated
Originated
Overhauled

Oversaw
Planned
Presided
Prioritized
Produced
Recommended
Reorganized
Replaced
Restored
Reviewed
Scheduled
Streamlined
Strengthened
Supervised
Terminated

Communication Skills

Addressed
Advertised
Arbitrated
Arranged
Articulated
Authored
Clarified
Collaborated
Communicated
Composed
Condensed
Conferred
Consulted
Contacted
Conveyed
Convinced
Corresponded
Debated
Defined
Described
Developed

Directed
Discussed
Drafted
Edited
Elicited
Empathised
Enlisted
Explained
Expressed
Formulated
Furnished
Incorporated
Influenced
Interacted
Interpreted
Interviewed
Involved
Joined
Lectured
Listened
Mediated
Moderated
Negotiated
Observed
Outlined
Participated
Persuaded
Presented
Promoted
Proposed
Publicized
Reconciled
Recruited
Referred
Reinforced
Reported
Resolved
Responded
Solicited
Specified

Spoke
Suggested
Summarized
Synthesized
Translated

Research Skills

Analysed
Clarified
Collected
Compared
Conducted
Critiqued
Detected
Determined
Diagnosed
Evaluated
Examined
Experimented
Explored
Extracted
Formulated
Gathered
Identified
Inspected
Interpreted
Interviewed
Invented
Investigated
Located
Measured
Organized
Researched
Searched
Solved
Summarized
Surveyed
Systematized
Tested

Teaching Skills

Adapted
Advised
Clarified
Coached
Communicated
Conducted
Coordinated

Critiqued
Developed
Enabled
Encouraged
Evaluated
Explained
Facilitated
Focused
Guided
Individualized
Informed
Instilled
Instructed
Motivated
Persuaded
Set Goals
Simulated
Stimulated
Taught
Tested
Trained
Transmitted
Tutored

Helping Skills

Adapted
Advocated
Aided
Answered
Assessed
Assisted
Clarified
Coached
Collaborated
Contributed
Cooperated
Counselled
Demonstrated
Educated
Encouraged
Ensured
Expedited
Facilitated
Familiarize
Insured
Intervened
Motivated
Provided
Referred

Rehabilitated
Presented
Resolved
Simplified
Supplied
Supported
Volunteered

Organisational and Management Skills

Approved
Arranged
Catalogued
Categorized
Charted
Classified
Coded
Collected
Compiled
Corresponded
Distributed
Executed
Filed
Generated
Implemented
Incorporated
Inspected
Logged
Maintained
Monitored
Obtained
Operated
Ordered
Organized
Prepared
Processed
Provided
Purchased
Recorded
Registered
Reserved
Responded
Reviewed
Routed
Scheduled
Screened
Set Up
Submitted

PORTFOLIO

2 PORTFOLIO

2.1 Motivational Questions

2.1.1 Why should we choose you?

Alternative Questions
- Tell me about your CV
- Tell me about yourself
- What will you bring to the specialty?

What interviewers are looking for

This is an extremely popular interview question and is designed to give you the opportunity to open up to the interviewers and tell them why you should be selected. The open nature of the question allows you to talk through your CV highlights and demonstrate your personality to the interviewers.

How to answer

Broad, open, background questions can seem daunting and are tricky to answer well. Remember the portfolio station is your time to summarise your most impressive achievements and it is important that you are enthusiastic about your accomplishments and provide your answers in a structured manner to help interviewers score you. Interviewers are not looking for a long, autobiographical journey through your CV but rather want to know your key selling points in each domain outlined by the person specification and consequently your suitability for selection into obstetrics and gynaecology.

The **CAMP** framework of Clinical, Academic, Management and Personal is a good way to create a coherent answer. Don't stick precisely to this order, instead put your achievements with the most impact first. Alternatively you may wish to structure your answer more closely to the person specification or the order in which you have laid out your CV. Any structure is fine provided it guides interviewers and prevents you from forgetting key achievements.
Try to keep each part to 2-3 minutes as time is limited and interviewers will begin to nod-off if you talk for too long!

Approach

Begin your answer confidently with a positive statement of your greatest achievement. You do not need to state that you should be chosen over other candidates but should present the interviewers with evidence of outstanding accomplishments that follow the person specification. Whatever achievements you select be sure to reflect upon them and say why they will make you a good colleague.
The next page contains some examples of achievements you may wish to use when structuring your answer.

Clinical	Academic
<ul><li>Log book summary</li><li>Clinical competence</li></ul>	<ul><li>Papers you have published</li><li>Postgraduate degrees awarded</li><li>Research undertaken</li><li>Teaching qualifications, courses and sessions</li></ul>
Management	Personal
<ul><li>Involvement with quality improvement</li><li>Rota organiser</li><li>Committee member</li><li>Organising events/course</li><li>Writing books</li><li>Updating guidelines</li></ul>	<ul><li>Personal strengths backed up by WBAs</li><li>Extracurricular achievements</li><li>Sports, musical instruments, etc.</li></ul>

Example

 "I am most proud of my logbook which I have cultivated in my current DGH. I have assisted with a list of over XX caesarean sections and XX diagnostic laparoscopies. I can close the abdominal layers with supervision, assess fetal positions for instrumental deliveries and perform perineal repairs. In addition I have been able to make management decisions assessing patients when on call, for example in the maternal assessment unit and early pregnancy unit. I have developed my skills in antenatal and gynaecology clinics to the point that I see patients independently. I will take these skills forward and continue to develop them in my role as an O&G trainee."

Exercise

 Write It Out

Write out an example answer with four paragraphs covering the **CAMP** structure. Use personal examples and link them to buzzwords and the person specification. Don't worry about it not being perfect first time, just do it and then come back and edit it so that you have a basic template for this common interview question.

TOP TIPS

✚ **Selling Yourself:** This can prove challenging as candidates do not wish to come off as overconfident or cocky. Rather use examples and feedback to demonstrate how good you are e.g. 'My 360 appraisal graded my communication skills as excellent'.

✚ **Be Positive and Sell, Sell, Sell:** Interviewers want to hear how great you are and it is important that you are not bashful or reserved when telling them about your achievements and why they should choose you. Turn everything into a positive and don't undersell yourself.

✚ **Be Personal:** Talking about generic things like 'I have leadership skills' will not score you as many points as using personal experiences for example 'I demonstrated my leadership skills managing a woman with a post-partum haemorrhage, I was the first to the scene and performed an ABC assessment followed by bimanual compression whilst directing other team members individually in the room. I learnt multiple things including…'

✚ **Mind Map:** Use a mind map or just jot down your main headings *(CAMP)* and then add in your own personal examples under each term. This will help you to remember all the things you have done and structure your answer under pressure.

PORTFOLIO

2.1.2 What is your greatest strength?

Alternative Questions

- What is your unique selling point?
- What are you most proud of?
- What makes you stand out from everyone else applying?
- What is the strongest area of your CV?
- What is your greatest personal strength?

What interviewers are looking for:

Your key selling points that make you suitable for obstetrics and gynaecology.
To establish whether your strengths are suitable for obstetrics and gynaecology.
To gain insight into your character and self-confidence.

How to answer

Everyone has strengths and weaknesses. To answer this question well and score maximum points it is not simply a case of reciting a list of as many strengths as possible but rather selecting a few of what you consider to be the strongest areas of your CV. Use examples from your CV to demonstrate that these strengths are proven and, most importantly, reflect on how they relate to obstetrics and gynaecology training.

> **Choose and reflect on a CV strength**
>
> **Strength**: Teaching
> **CV Example**: Attaining a postgraduate certificate in teaching on contraceptive methods.
> **Reflection**: The audience preferred interactive teaching to power point teaching. Spontaneous discussions were effective, lots of individuals were keen to reflect on their experiences with patients and I developed discussions around this.

How to avoid sounding arrogant

Most medics are bad at selling themselves and are worried about sounding overconfident when asked to talk about their achievements. While it is true that appearing arrogant will likely go down poorly with interviewers under-selling your achievements is equally as detrimental.

An easy way to get around this problem is to put examples from your CV at the centre of the discussion rather than yourself.

For example a candidate who says:

'I am excellent at communicating with patients' may come across as arrogant. Whereas a candidate who says:

'My greatest strength has been highlighted through my 360 degree feedback where my communication skills were rated as excellent by 10 separate raters' This not only provides evidence behind the claim but also puts the comparative term 'excellent' on the communication skills.

In essence rather than saying you are excellent it is your communication skills that are excellent and others have said this not just you.

Approach

You can structure this answer using **CAMP** or using a clinical and an extra-curricular achievement.

You might also like to use an umbrella term such as 'teaching' or 'research' as your strength and then go on to elaborate about individual papers, degrees, teaching sessions etc. that you have given.

PORTFOLIO

Clinical:	Extracurricular:
• Publication	• Marathon
• Organising conference	• Triathlon
• Updating guidelines	• Team sports
• Postgraduate degree	• Teaching yourself language/
• 360 appraisal	instrument etc

Example

 "I have many things that I am proud of including writing medical text-books, completing an MSc and receiving excellent feedback from patients and peers. But the two things I consider my greatest achievements are my organisational skills and my teaching skills. I demonstrated both of these when I organised a regional teaching day for foundation doctors which required me to locate a venue, arrange speakers, set a programme for the day and teach on practical workshops. 30 foundation doctors attended the teaching day with consultants lecturing and running surgical skills workshops. This experience will prove invaluable when teaching juniors and when organising my time between gaining operative experience and improving my CV during obstetrics and gynaecology training."

PORTFOLIO

TOP TIPS

✚ **Selling:** The key to this question *(as with many others)* is that even if the examples you give are fairly ordinary you need to make them sound like they are fantastic achievements that you are proud of.

✚ **Reflect:** Remember that points are awarded for why the achievement is so special and how it relates to surgery. Make sure you reflect on the underlying skills and values and try to use the person specification to relate back to obstetrics and gynaecology.

2.1.3   What is your biggest weakness?

Alternative Questions
- What can you improve?
- How can your CV be improved?
- What is the weakest area of your CV?
- 'X' is not very good on your CV. What have you done about it?

What interviewers are looking for

To see how you react when presented with a direct, negative question or state-ment (essentially being put under pressure).
To ascertain your insight and self-awareness for areas of improvement.
To identify areas for improvement and to understand why that area is weak.

How to answer

Talking about weaknesses is tricky. When presented with a negative question under pressure some candidates may panic or may even fall into a depression where they agree with the interviewers that an area of their CV is particularly weak and talk themselves out of a job!
The key to this question is turning your weakness into a positive and leaving the interviewers with a feeling that you have identified an area lacking in your CV and have then done something about it.

Approach

Unless asked specifically about a personal weakness always try to use an area of your CV or professional weakness that can be easily be improved. In the unlikely event that a personal weakness is asked for try not to pick anything too serious and choose something that can be easily corrected.
You can structure your answer in a similar way to 'your greatest strength' and after mentioning the weakness reflect on how it is in fact a positive.

 From Across The Table: Interviewer's Tip

Don't do as several candidates have done in the past and say 'I have no weaknesses' as you will not score highly and interviewers are likely to make your life very difficult for the remainder of the station. Also try not to inject any humour as one candidate did when he simply replied 'Kryptonite'.

Example: CV weakness

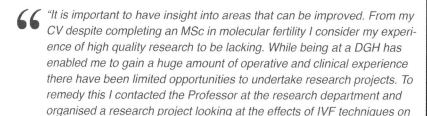 *"It is important to have insight into areas that can be improved. From my CV despite completing an MSc in molecular fertility I consider my experience of high quality research to be lacking. While being at a DGH has enabled me to gain a huge amount of operative and clinical experience there have been limited opportunities to undertake research projects. To remedy this I contacted the Professor at the research department and organised a research project looking at the effects of IVF techniques on obstetric outcomes."*

Or a personal weakness that is relatable:

"I have high standards and like efficiency I therefore get frustrated when there are delays in collecting patients and dead time between surgical cases. I highlighted this as an area for improvement and found that it is important to take a step back, let staff do their jobs and see if there are practical ways to improve efficiency. I have recently set up an audit looking at theatre staffing levels for elective caesareans as this was one of the major causes in list delays."

PORTFOLIO

TOP TIPS

➕ **Choosing a Weakness**: Don't choose anything too bad, rather select something that is relatable and can be improved.

➕ **Don't Dwell On It:** Touch briefly on the weakness and then quickly move the interview towards more positive things.

➕ **Identification and Initiative:** Points will be awarded for both identifying a weakness and then demonstrating that you have used your initiative and done something to remedy or improve that weakness. Examples might include finding a mentor, undertaking an audit or research project, attending a course or simply reading up on a topic.

➕ **Follow On Questions:** Be prepared for interviewers to push you for more areas of weakness. One candidate was asked for four further examples of areas that could be improved!

2.1.4	Why are you applying for Obstetrics and Gynaecology?

Alternative Questions
- Why do you want to be an obs gynae doctor?
- O&G training is long. Why bother?
- Why have you applied for this post?
- What do you like most about this specialty?

What interviewers are looking for

Interviewers want to know that you fully understand what the job entails, that you have researched the entry and selection criteria and that you are enthusiastic for a career in O&G.

How to answer

This is a motivational question and is again open and broad in scope. As with all open, motivational questions you need to present a succinct, focused answer covering key points that relate to the person specification while highlighting your understanding of what the role entails.

Thus you should not only explain your own motivations for applying but also imply why you are a suitable candidate for selection.

Having done your research and having read the introductory chapter of this book you should have a basic idea of what interviewers are looking for and you should give your answer in an enthusiastic manner. Remember the interviewers are O&G surgeons who (hopefully) enjoy their job and you should too.

Approach

Your answer may wish to utilise the **CAMP** structure or a variant such as just personal and academic. Alternatively you may also wish to use a chronological, story-based framework to guide your answer recounting when and why you first decided upon a career in O&G and what you subsequently did to make that a reality.

Whatever reasons you have for doing O&G make sure that they are personal and you are enthusiastic. The table on the next page summarises some key aspects of the specialty.

From Across The Table: Interviewer's Tip

Remember that it is not just what you say but also how you say it. Smile and be enthusiastic about doing obstetrics and gynaecology as a career. Interviewers will be able to spot candidates who are not convincing and it is nice for interviewers to hear how great their day job can be.

Clinical	Academic
Challenging, wide range of subspecialties Patient mix (young vs old, well vs unwell) elective and emergency procedures Able to make immediate impact to patients' lives Enjoy operating and receiving immediate feedback from trainers Be involved in prevention, treatment and follow-up of patients Interventions can rapidly and dramatically improve quality of life for patients	Evidence-based approach, strong research component, strong interface with technology, industry and MDT. Opportunity to teach practical skills and learn from peers and experienced O&G surgeons, lifelong learning continual advances.

Management	Personal
Opportunity to improve care on a wider scale Develop organisational skills such as arranging lists, organising teaching or rotas	Personal experience of surgery Relative with illness Enjoy fast-pace Enjoy pressure Enjoy practical skills Find it fun and challenging and it helps people

Example

The below example uses a combination of the **CAMP** framework and a chronological structure to convey both motivation and suitability for selection.

 "During medical school I enjoyed my O&G placements the most out of all the specialties. In particular I enjoyed the practical nature of the subject, from assessing fetal position, performing USS and undertaking surgery. I found the surgery to be diverse ranging from minimal access surgery to laparotomies and caesarean sections. I also enjoyed the medical spectrum associated with diagnosis, for example interpreting the physiology behind an abnormal CTG and assessing patients in assessment units. I subsequently set up an O&G society for students and upon graduation selected foundation rotations with O&G and researched what was required for selection and progression in surgery. I attended BSS and ALSO courses and enjoyed learning key surgical principles and pathology required to pass the MRCOG Part 1. My passion for both teaching and research together with my ability to work under pressure and enjoyment of technical skills make me determined to progress through O&G training and onto higher training."

PORTFOLIO

2.1.5   What do you like least about the specialty?

Alternative Questions
- Tell me some negatives about a career in O&G?
- Is O&G always fun?
- Do all O&G trainees enjoy their jobs?

What interviewers are looking for

Interviewers want to know that you are aware of the potential negative aspects of a career in O&G. They are looking for insight and awareness so that potential difficulties do not come as a surprise to you if you are selected.

How to answer

Like the question about weaknesses this is all about making sure that you show that you have made an attempt to do something about the thing that you dislike. Choose an example that all O&G trainees might find tedious and remember to give both a personal example of your experiences of this together with some suggestions to improve or ways to deal with the problem.

> #### ⌒ From Across The Table: Interviewer's Tip
>
> Do not come across as too negative and try to avoid making it personal. This is not an opportunity to express your views on the decline of the NHS simply highlight a negative and move on.

Approach

You may not have been immersed in an O&G specialty to know all the minor bugbears. Think about what registrars or consultants complain about (remember medics love to complain!). Some common examples are listed below:

- The European Working Time Directive limiting training opportunities and creating shift-patterns. For example at ST1 level the training MATRIX requires you to have experience in fetal blood sampling, manual removal of placentas, caesarean sections, instrumental deliveries *(both forceps and ventouse)* and others. The EWTD limits your opportunities to achieve these goals.
- The decline of the traditional O&G 'firm' due to the EWTD and training reforms with doctors more frequently rotating between jobs.
- The role of management and service provision in limiting time and opportunities for training.
- The length and cost of O&G training. It costs to sit the MRCOG Part One and to attend compulsory courses such as basic practical skills. There are also other courses that are beneficial for your training, for example on instrumental deliveries. These courses are all expensive.

Example

 "Because I very much enjoy O&G there are certain things that I have found frustrating. Influence of industry, finance and management on patient operations and training."

The above is a good answer but you will need to expand on it and reflect if you wish to score maximum marks.

Better example with reflection

 "From my experience patient surgeries may be delayed if the correct kit has not been ordered or is not on the shelf and trainees are increasingly asked by management to provide service provision on non-teaching lists rather than be learning from experienced surgeons."

 "I think that trainees should be more involved with local management and liaising with industry/scrub staff to ensure training is maximised and kit is available. I have organised a quality improvement audit looking at delays to theatre..."

2.1.6 | What are your short or long term goals?

Alternative Questions
- Where do you see yourself in 5 or 10 years time?
- What kind of O&G doctor would you like to be?

What interviewers are looking for

Interviewers want to know that you have a career plan and have thought about what you will be doing during your O&G training years. In years ST6-ST7 you will be undertaking speciality modules of interest. It might be worth considering where you interests could potentially lie or an area that you are considering getting more experience in. Examples include labour ward, urogynaecology, fertility, minimal access surgery and gynaeoncology.

How to answer

This questions looks at your planning and commitment to the specialty. This is an opportunity to highlight projects you may have started such as higher degrees or research and talk about how you plan on completing them. Think about what stage of surgical training you will be at. In 5 years you will be a registrar and in 10 years you will be on fellowship or will have just started as a consultant.

PORTFOLIO

Approach

Begin with short term goals and use the CAMP framework to structure your answer: what projects are you doing, what degrees are you doing, what operative experience are you aiming for.

Structure your long-term goals in a similar fashion. Will you be on fellowship, what kind of hospital will you be working in, what specialty will you be working in, where will you be in your personal life.

Example

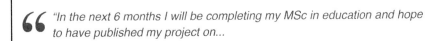

"In the next 6 months I will be completing my MSc in education and hope to have published my project on...

In the future I would like to be a consultant specialising in minimal access surgery in a teaching hospital..."

Exercise

 Write out your career goals

Write a short summary of where you see yourself in 6-months, 1 year and 5 years time. Be specific and if you plan to sit an exam or undertake some research write these down.

2.2 | Situational Ability Questions

2.2.1 | How would you describe your communication skills?

Alternative Questions
- Are you a good communicator?
- How have your communication skills made a difference?
- How would colleagues describe your communication skills

What interviewers are looking for

Interviewers are looking for specific examples that demonstrate good communication skills. They also want to see insight into the importance of communication skills and how they can be developed.

How to answer

Communication skills can be difficult to quantify, luckily your WBAs, patient feedback and teaching feedback provide plenty of ammunition to prove how good your communication skills are.

If you have struggled with communication skills but have done something about it such as attending a course and shown improvement this is also a good example.

Approach

Rather than simply talking about your 'communication skills' try to give specific examples of communication elements such as:

- Explaining a procedure/diagnosis
- Breaking bad news
- Active listening to a patient
- Showing empathy
- Dealing with an angry relative
- Negotiating an urgent scan or investigation

Use either examples from your portfolio or short work-based examples of your communication skills in action. For the later the STAR framework of situation, task, action, result/reflection can be used to structure your explanation of how your communication skills led to a result and how you reflected on this.

Example

"I believe that I have excellent communication skills as demonstrated by my 360 degree feedback and when effectively consenting patients for surgery, discussing treatment options in clinic and giving regular teach-

PORTFOLIO

ing sessions to large audiences. Specific examples can be shown in my portfolio such as feedback from a recent obstetrics and gynaecology career day that I organised for medical students at which I gave lectures covering the key obstetric emergencies."

TOP TIPS

 Selling Yourself: This can often prove challenging as candidates do not wish to come off as overconfident or cocky. Rather use examples and feedback to demonstrate how good you are. E.g. 'My 360 appraisal graded my communication skills as excellent'

PORTFOLIO

2.2.2	Is empathy important for O&G trainees?

Alternative Questions

- Give an example when you showed empathy to a patient.
- How have your communication skills influenced a patient's management?
- Tell me about a case that affected you emotionally

What interviewers want

All doctors need to possess empathy to be able to appreciate the emotions of patients that they are treating. Interviewers are looking for evidence from your work-based assessments if possible and an example of a case where you were able to empathise with a patient in a way that impacted their care in a positive way.

How to answer

You should consider this question an extension of your communication skills answer with focus specifically on building rapport and empathising with a patient. Think of a time that you have used your communication skills to help a patient or of a case where you felt particularly for a patient. This could be as simple as putting an anxious patient at ease about an operation or breaking bad news to family members in a supportive way.

✑ From Across The Table: Interviewer's Tip

Story Telling: Use personal examples that tell the interviewers a story. This will be more engaging than listing things and will also demonstrate insight into patient care.

Approach

Select an example that demonstrates your communication skills and use the **STAR** framework reflecting on how your empathy improved things for the patient.

Example

 "A 48-year-old lady with menorrhagia asked to speak with me as the patient and her husband were unhappy with her care during a weekend on-call period. She had a large fibroid but no other abnormality on ultrasound scan and was refusing to take pain relief or tranexamic acid. I spoke with them in a quiet side room and asked a nurse to hold my bleep and inform me only if there was an emergency. I could tell from their body language and tone that they were unhappy and I used empathy and active listening to establish that they felt they did not understand what was going on. I then succinctly conveyed the diagnosis and treatment plan in an understandable way and encouraged the patient to trial tranexamic to facilitate her recovery. I also explained that she would be followed up by the gynaecology team. I know this was effective as the nursing staff noted that the family were happy with the outcome and the patient was discharged the following day. I received a thank you letter from the patient saying that I helped her to understand things and previously she had just felt like a nuisance and was frightened. The card is in my portfolio."

2.2.3	Are you a good team player?

Alternative Questions

- Give an example of your teamwork skills
- Do you work better alone or as part of a team?
- Tell me about a team you have been in
- What is teamwork?

What interviewers are looking for

Teamwork is an essential part of O&G training, whether you are in theatre with the scrub and anaesthetic team, part of labour ward or simply on the ward with the nurses, midwives and other SHOs. Interviewers want to know that you understand the core components of being a team player and work well both alone and as part of a team.

How to answer

Your answer should convey three key facts:

- You are able to communicate and work effectively with others
- You are able to appreciate the roles and viewpoints of other team members
- You are able to make a valuable individual contribution to the team

Use specific, work-based examples that can be backed-up with evidence from your work-based assessments to highlight effective teams that you have been a part of. Remember to reflect on the experience and to focus on aspects of a good team player (see box).

Qualities of a good team player:

- Understands their role and how it fits in with the overall team.
- Is reliable, consistent, works hard, seeks help appropriately, takes initiative
- Treats others with respect
- Appreciates the role of others, approachable, responds to requests, allows others to perform their role, offer support when required
- Flexible and able to compromise
- Can adapt to changes, can consider different viewpoints, can compromise with other team members
- Communicates and listens
- Expresses thoughts clearly, proposes solutions not problems to the team, understands and listens to other views, accepts and acts on criticisms and feedback

---

Approach

The **STAR** framework may be employed to structure your answer.

Example

 "I am an excellent team player as outlined by my 360 appraisals and the results of projects such as...

Situation: *Writing a paper/book*
Task: *I was responsible for co-authors and contributors and was required to motivate my peers while delegating work*
Action: *I was supportive and flexible if contributors were struggling with their workload. I listened to contributors and acted upon suggestions and improvements that they felt would help the text.*

Result/Reflection: *This experience impressed upon me the importance of maintaining good rapport with people and the paper has now been published."*

TOP TIPS

 Teamwork: Think about what makes an effective team and how teams that you have been part of have functioned.

2.2.4 Are you a good leader?

Alternative Questions
- Tell us about your leadership experience
- What makes a good leader?
- Are you more of a leader or a manager?

PORTFOLIO

What interviewers are looking for

It is important that you can not only be a team member but can also lead a team. Interviewers are looking for examples of how you have led projects and people and the subsequent results.

How to answer

The difference between leadership and management can be tricky to define and certain aspects of each seem to overlap. Essentially leaders are concerned with using initiative to drive people towards a result that changes current practice. Managers are more focused on organising people to maintain current standards. Leaders change, managers maintain.

Leaders	Managers
Leaders drive a group forward to implement change. Leaders make decisions, organise and motivate team members	Managers organise a group to ensure the status-quo is maintained. Managers organise team members, ensure they meet deadlines and prioritise tasks

You will have been involved in situations that have required both leadership and management. These may be limited having come from F2 so try to interpret the question as 'How will you become a good leader' and discuss the qualities of good leaders you have worked with, examples of your own leadership and how you will develop these skills in obstetrics and gynaecology training.

Leadership Roles:

- Creating a teaching programme
- Writing a book or book chapter with contributors
- Leading a cardiac arrest call
- Captaining a sports team
- Leading a fundraising drive
- Leading a quality improvement project

PORTFOLIO

Approach

To answer this question think about people you consider to be good leaders and use personal examples to illustrate the qualities that they possess.
Use the **STAR** framework to help you structure your example answer. Ensure that you use personal examples of how you have led projects and utilise any work based assessments or feedback on your leadership skills. Remember to reflect on your experiences and mention how you will develop your leadership skills during O&G training.

Example

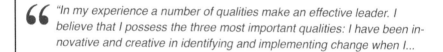 *"In my experience a number of qualities make an effective leader. I believe that I possess the three most important qualities: I have been innovative and creative in identifying and implementing change when I...*

I then demonstrated passion and enthusiasm in encouraging others to become involved with the project by... Finally I am able to develop results and complete tasks. I have shown this with the positive feedback and strong outcomes of..."

TOP TIPS

Leadership: If you are struggling think about the best leader that you know in or out of work. What characteristics do they possess that make others listen and follow them? You may also wish to look at the action words section of The Basics chapter of this book to help you think about words and actions that imply leadership qualities.

2.2.5	Tell me about your management skills

Alternative Questions
- Are you a good manager?
- What makes a good manager?
- How do you manage people?
- Tell me about a project you have managed

What interviewers are looking for

All O&G trainees must possess management skills in order to maintain standards. Interviewers are looking for an understanding of a trainee's role as a manager, what this involves and examples of how you have demonstrated management skills.

How to answer

Managers are concerned with handling people and colleagues in order to meet set standards. Their skills are mainly organisational and are centred around analysing problems and communicating with people to maintain and achieve set goals.

Most interviewees (even at ST3 interviews) find management the most challenging area of their CV to fill. This is partly due to the ambiguous definition and partly due to perceived lack of exposure to management opportunities.

Example management roles:
- Sitting on a committee
- Organising a rota
- Quality improvement

Approach

The **STAR** framework can be used to structure your answer. Think about when you have organised and managed people or tasks.

Example

"During my O&G F2 placement I was tasked with organising the SHO rota for the F2s in order to ensure it was compliant with working hours and allowed all of the team to take annual leave within the allotted time. Feedback from my supervising consultant demonstrated my strong management skills as I was able to effectively communicate with the other F2s and prioritise leave requests while analysing and organising each SHOs shifts to maintain adequate ward cover and thus patient safety. I will continue to develop my management skills by becoming more involved with committee roles at local and regional level to help maintain standards of training."

2.2.6	Are you a good teacher?

Alternative Questions
- What makes a good teacher?
- What feedback have you had on teaching sessions given?
- Are you interested in medical education?
- What objective evidence do you have that demonstrates your teaching ability?

What interviewers are looking for

Trainees in O&G must possess a strong academic background and teaching and training future trainees has always been vital to the apprenticeship model of O&G training. Interviewers want evidence of teaching that you have been involved with together with feedback and understanding of the importance of teaching and the various methods of learning and delivering teaching.

How to answer

This open question may seem difficult to answer at first glance.
Summarise your teaching experience and use specific feedback from sessions given to demonstrate that you are a good teacher. The qualities of a good teacher can be fairly subjective depending on learning style.
The key to this question is to think of the best teacher you have had and elaborate on the qualities they possessed.

Qualities of a Good Teacher:

- Enthusiastic
- Experienced
- Involves student
- Listens to student
- Understands different learning styles
- Leading a quality improvement project

Make sure you finish the question by emphasising that you possess these qualities and back the claim up with evidence from your work-based assessments. This is also a good time to talk about any teaching degrees, courses or feedback you have.

Approach

The **STAR** framework should be utilised to structure your personal example. Focus on some of the qualities that you consider good teachers to possess and make sure you try to summarise the best teaching projects that you have been involved with.

Examples of Teaching:

- Undertaking a higher teaching degree
- Medical student teaching
- Departmental teaching
- Organising a teaching course
- Creating an e-learning resource

Example

 "Having completed a postgraduate certificate in medical education I could tell you many generic characteristics outlined by studies such as setting goals, creating a teaching plan, defining learning styles or respecting students however from my personal experiences the three most important characteristics are enthusiasm, being a role model and reflecting on feedback. I have demonstrated these when..."

PORTFOLIO

2.2.7 Tell me about your best audit

Alternative Questions
- What is your experience of audit?
- What do you understand by the meaning of an audit?
- What audits have you completed?
- What quality improvement projects have you been involved with?
- How have you improved patient care in your hospital?
- What is your most recent/current audit project?

What the interviewers are looking for

Quality improvement and maintaining patient safety through regular audit are a vital part of medicine. Interviewers want to know you have completed an audit cycle and have experience of the importance of audit together with the difficulties associated with ensuring standards are maintained even after the audit cycle has completed.

How to answer

This is a chance to talk about the audit that you are most proud of.
In preparing for this question make sure you know data for all of your audits included in your application even those completed a number of years ago. Also make sure you know where the audit is in your portfolio in case the interviewers have difficulty finding it.

> **Audit Definition**: An audit is a systematic quality improvement tool comparing current practices with set standards to maintain quality of patient care and outcomes.
>
> Audits are part of clinical governance and are important to patients, hospitals and doctors.
>
> - They maintain standards and outcomes in the healthcare setting.
> - They help maintain patient safety.
> - They help hospitals identify areas for improvement and help them meet standards.
> - They train junior doctors to be analytical and improve their management skills.
> - Data collected can be shared with other trusts to implement change on a larger scale.

Approach

Structure your answer by giving some background as to why it was important, the criteria for audit, the change implemented and the outcomes. You can use the **STAR** framework if you wish but having a structure that matches a standard audit proposal may be help show interviewers you have an understanding of the audit process.

Example

Background: "My trust had recently introduced guidelines for elective caesarean section enhanced recovery programmes. Some of the anaesthetists had noted that there was a difference between the individual O&G surgeons. My Consultant was keen for the department to be utilising the guidelines properly. It interested me as I had little experience of enhanced recovery and gave me the opportunity to look at the current literature, which demonstrated significant results."

Criteria: "Elective caesarean sections meet local guidelines using nutrition, mobilisation, early catheter removal and thromboprophylaxis'.
The audit identified that catheters were often late to be removed post operatively and the administration of LMWH was often delayed. There was poor documentation in the surgical operation note as to a patient's suitability for enhanced recovery."

Implementing change: "Education and implementation of a proforma"

Outcome: "The average inpatient stay reduced from 3.2 to 2.1 days post ELUSCS. Reducing bed costs (£225/day). Currently doing a re-audit looking at patient satisfaction scores."

TOP TIPS

✚ **Audit Summary:** It is a good idea to create a single A4 sheet summarising each of your audit projects using the subheadings above. This has two purposes; to remind you of the key points and facts of each audit and to make the audits easier to find within your portfolio.

✚ **Be Specific:** Remember to re-read all your audits. The above summary sheet will help with this but you can deflect difficult interview questions by ensuring you know specific facts such as the number of patients in a study, the timings of the study, the outcome improvement figures and where the outcomes are *(have they fallen back)* now.

2.2.8	Tell me about your research

Alternative Questions
- Tell me about the research project you are most proud of
- What is your most recent/current research project?
- Tell me about your publications
- What research have you been involved with?

What Interviewers are looking for

Research helps to advance O&G surgical techniques and principles and it is vital that any interventions offered to patients are evidence-based with documented, well-researched benefits, Interviewers are looking for knowledge of the importance of research, how research should be conducted, types of research and active involvement in a research project.

How to answer

This is an opportunity to be enthusiastic about your postgraduate degrees, publications and research projects. If you have little research experience or no publications talk about a current project that you are undertaking. Whatever you mention make sure you know where it is in your portfolio and all the data around it as follow up questions may catch you out.

PORTFOLIO

> **Research Definition**: Research is a systematic process to answer a question aiming to create new standards of care, helping to establish best practice.

Research can be thought of as being important to patients, hospital and doctors.

Patients: Advances Surgical Techniques and Patient Care
Research advances surgery and patient care by identifying new knowledge and treatments that benefit patients.

Hospitals: Improves Hospital Reputation and Funding
Research helps units and trusts to improve their reputation and secure funding.

Doctors: Improves Knowledge of Researchers
Research helps O&G trainees and Consultants to develop their understanding of conditions and pathologies, to back up their decisions with evidence based medicine and improves transferable skills such as analysis, problem-solving and organisation.

Approach

You should structure your answer as you would a research abstract with background, methods, results and conclusions. Alternatively if you are in the process of conducting research you may wish to describe the specific steps you have achieved thus far such as writing a funding proposal, identify a research question, setting a null hypothesis, calculating the study power or applying for ethics approval.

Example

"I have successfully completed two research projects and am currently undertaking a third. The research I am most proud of is a study of.... published in Injury. The study look at...and concluded that... I have also completed an MSc in... and am currently at the data collection stage for a study looking at..."

TOP TIPS

➕ **Selling Yourself:** This can often prove challenging as candidates do not wish to come off as overconfident or cocky. Rather use examples and feedback to demonstrate how good you are e.g. 'I successfully received funding for my research project'

➕ **Be Specific:** Similar to the audit section above make sure that you know all the facts and figures related to your research.

2.2.9	Probity: Tell me about a mistake you have made

Alternative Questions
- Tell me about a time you have shown integrity
- Have you had any operative complications?
- Have you received a complaint?

What interviewers are looking for

All doctors must demonstrate probity and honesty as outlined by the GMC. Interviewers want to know that you are honest and can take responsibility for any mistakes you may have made.

How to answer

Everyone has made a mistake or had an operative complication and if you have not you will do in the future. The key aspect is that any mistake or complaint should be acknowledge, investigated and then treated as a learning point to see if current practices can be improved. Select a mistake that was not serious but has a good learning point attached. As with all 'negative' questions do not get phased but rather see this as an opportunity to turn the question into a positive. Make sure you are honest in your account and remember that the most important part is reflecting and acting on the outcome.

Approach

The **STAR** framework can be used to answer this question. Remember that interviewers may push you for more mistakes and learning points so ensure you have a few good examples prepared.

Example

 "During a busy oncall period I was asked by a ward nurse to mark a patient who had been consented but not marked and was with porters waiting to go to theatre. I quickly read the notes and consent form and explained to the patient I needed to mark his arm. He put forward his left arm towards me and I went to mark the arm with the marker before quickly realising that it was actually the opposite elbow that was to be operated on. I apologised to the patient and marked the correct arm. My mistake would have delayed his surgery and could have led to a never event of wrong site surgery. Subsequently I looked up the incidence of wrong site surgery (1/10000) and now ensure that I calmly look at imaging, patients notes, consent form and ask the patient prior to marking the surgical site."

PORTFOLIO

2.2.10	Risk: Are you involved with risk management?

Alternative Questions
- How do doctors manage risk?
- When did you last perform a risk assessment?
- How are you involved in maintaining patient safety?

What interviewers are looking for

Interviewers want to see that candidates have knowledge and awareness of risk and patient safety. All doctors are involved in assessing risk and interviewers want personal examples of your involvement.

How to answer

This can seem like a fairly ambiguous question and requires some understanding of what risk management actually is. Risk management is one of the pillars of clinical governance.

Risk Management is a large topic in obstetrics and gynaecology. You should be aware of the risk management department for O&G and familiarise yourself with some important cases. You should be aware of the Montgomery case and never events. An example of a never event is leaving a vaginal swab in situ.

Risk can be divided into: risk to patients, risk to staff and risk to organisation.

Risk to patients: is minimised by adhering to national standards and ensuring that the standards are maintained. In essence clinical audit helps to minimise patient risk and maintain patient safety.

Risk to staff: is minimised by ensuring staff are immunised and are aware of work-place risks by completing mandatory trust training for skills such as manual handling and conflict resolution.

Risk to organisation: is minimised by reducing risk to the above two and by ensuring frameworks are in place to deal with organisational issues such as filling empty rota slots with locums, securing confidential data and maintaining workplace safety.

By default you will have been to and possibly taught at a departmental induction for staff and colleagues, which minimises staff risk. You will have undertaken a clinical audit to maintain patient safety and are involved in risk management on a daily basis when assessing and prioritising patients.

Approach

The **STAR** framework can be used to answer this question. Choose a personal example and remember to reflect on what you learned relating to risk.

Example

 "I am regularly involved in risk management, a particular example is when I am assessing a patient for theatre. I identify risk factors in patients, such as a high ASA grade, a raised BMI or previous abdominal surgery in patients having laparoscopic surgery. At the start of the operation I take part in the WHO surgical checklist to ensure that set criteria are met before the patient is operated upon, for example I am always aware of the placental site prior to a caesarean section starting, as well as the patients blood group incase cord blood gases are required. Finally I am regularly involved in audits and have recently undertaken an audit of correct swab use on labour ward. All women with swabs in situ should have a green band on their wrist. I undertook an audit to check that this standard was being maintained."

2.2.11 Judgement: Can you work under pressure?

Alternative Questions
- How do you cope with stress?
- Surgery is stressful. Will you cope?
- Give us an example of a stressful situation you have been in?

What the interviewers want

Interviewers want to know that you can function effectively in high-pressure environments such as trauma calls and emergencies. Interviewers want evidence of experience of working under pressure and personal strategies to both identify stress and to cope with high-pressure, stressful environments.

High Pressure Situations
- Obstetric emergency call e.g. shoulder dystocia, post-partum haemorrhage, cord prolapse, unexpected breech, fetal bradycardia
- Unwell patient, e.g sepsis in the postnatal patient
- On call covering multiple patients
- Acting up, your registrar is busy in a caesarean with the consultant and a patient has just arrived with a large antenatal bleed
- Covering a sick colleague, low staff
- Assisting in a life-saving operation eg hysterectomy for large PPH
- Dealing with an emergency, cardiac arrest for suspected pulmonary embolism
- Difficult/angry patient or relative

PORTFOLIO

How to answer

Regardless of how the above question is asked interviewers want a personal example of a high-pressure, stressful situation that you have identified, experienced, what you did, how you coped with it and what you learned that you will take forward into obstetrics and gynaecology training.

> **Coping Strategies:**
>
> - Prioritising tasks
> - Seeking help
> - Delegating work
> - Remaining calm and thinking
> - Taking a step back and assessing
> - Having insight into when you are stressed
> - Staying healthy, taking breaks and resting

Approach

The **STAR** framework can be used to answer this question. Remember that interviewers may push you for more mistakes and learning points so ensure you have a few good examples prepared.

Example

 "I am able to identify potentially stressful situations and work under pressure to a high level as demonstrated by 360 feedback. When working on a busy medical admissions unit overnight with a team member down I was tasked with clerking in over 40 new medical admissions with just the on call registrar. The registrar was also dealing with sick ward patients meaning that I was often left alone on the unit. I identified this as a stressful situation and prioritised the sickest patients to be triaged first while ensure that I took breaks when possible and kept hydrated. When both the registrar and myself began to get overwhelmed by the number of unwell new admissions we contacted the on call consultant who came in to help with the workload. Between the three of us we were able to safely staff the unit overnight and maintain patient safety. Looking after myself while prioritising and seeking help when required will prove an invaluable experience when dealing with surgical emergencies especially in situations where either the registrar or myself are also required to be operating in theatre"

2.3 | Specific Questions

2.3.1 | Academic

What is an audit?

An audit is a systematic quality improvement tool comparing current practices with set standards to maintain quality of patient care and outcomes.

What is the audit cycle?

Clinical audit has a number of defined stages. Stages five and re-audit below encompass closure of the audit loop.

- Stage 1: Identify the problem or issue
- Stage 2: Define criteria & standards
- Stage 3: Data collection
- Stage 4: Compare performance with criteria and standards
- Stage 5: Implementing change
- Re-audit: Sustaining improvements

Why is audit important?

Audits are part of clinical governance and are important to patients, hospitals and doctors.

- They maintain standards and outcomes in the healthcare setting.
- They help maintain patient safety.
- They help hospitals identify areas for improvement and help them meet standards.
- They train junior doctors to be analytical and improve their management skills.
- Data collected can be shared with other trusts to implement change on a larger scale.

What problems have you encountered with audits that you have conducted?

Try to use a personal example if possible. An audit that you didn't complete would be acceptable provided you say why.

Problems:

- Local process and may not be easily transferable
- Junior doctors rotate through departments meaning sustainability is poor
- Finding solutions to the problems found can be difficult
- Suggested change may not always be popular with staff or create more work for staff
- Creates more work for busy junior doctors

PORTFOLIO

Example

> "I undertook an audit into ward-based VTE thromboprophylaxis to ensure that drug charts were correctly completed. After successfully completing the audit loop we were able to improve VTE prescribing. Frustratingly 6-months later standards had dropped down to their previous level and sustainability was tricky due to the junior doctors rotating and no, one person taking a lead. We therefore assigned a role to one of the senior nursing staff to ensure levels are maintained. This in itself does create more work but does ensure that standards are maintained."

What is the difference between research and audit? Is an audit research?

Clinical audit is 'a quality improvement process that seeks to improve patient care and outcomes through systematic review of care against explicit criteria and the implementation of change'.
Research is a one-off, systematic and organised way to find answers to questions. Research does not check whether you are complying with standards, instead its aim is to create new knowledge and new standards.
In essence research helps to establish best practice while audit ensures that best practice is carried out.

What do you understand about levels of evidence in research? What level of evidence is your research project?

Oxford Centre for Evidence-Based Medicine (EBM)

I RCT/Meta-analysis
II Cohort Study
III Case-Control Study
IV Case Series
V Expert Opinion

Should research be compulsory? Who should do research?

This is a somewhat loaded question as the person specification scores you on research completed.

The question wants you to give an argument for and against. You do not need to reach a firm conclusion but rather appreciate that research is important but it is not for everybody. This is also an opportunity to talk about your own research and move the interview along.

Example

> "Research is an important part of medical practise and part of clinical governance. Not every trainee has access to research centres and many in DGHs struggle to organise good research projects. Not everyone will

PORTFOLIO

want to take time out to complete a higher degree but the option is there for those who do. Personally I enjoy research and have completed 3 projects..."

Describe how you would answer a research question

If you have set up your own research project use this as a personal example and comment on the steps involved and difficulties encountered.

The basic steps are outlined below:

- Literature review,
- Find supervisor with experience,
- Null hypothesis,
- Primary aims,
- Power and sample size calculation with statistician,
- Ethics committee approval,
- Cost analysis and funding approval if necessary,
- Start recruiting patients,
- Collect data,
- Statistical analysis,
- Conclude,
- Write-up,
- Publish,
- Present.

What are validity and reliability?

Validity: is comprehensiveness – does it measure what it intends to measure?

Reliability: is the error in a measurement tool or its consistency

What are sensitivity and specificity?

Sensitivity: measures the proportion of actual positives which are correctly identified as such (e.g. the percentage of sick people who are correctly identified as having the condition)

Specificity: measures the proportion of negatives which are correctly identified as such (e.g. the percentage of healthy people who are correctly identified as not having the condition)

How do you decide if a treatment is worth implementing?

All treatments should have level one research proving that they are effective in their outcome. They should be evidence-based. Once a treatment has been proven to be effective it should undergo a cost-analysis to ensure that it is practical to offer it to patients over other treatments. In a cost-effectiveness analysis, the benefits of a treatment are expressed in non-monetary terms related to health, such as symptom-free days, heart attacks avoided, deaths avoided or life years gained (that is, the number of years by which the intervention extends life). Cost-effectiveness analysis assesses the cost of achieving the same benefit by different means.

What is a gold standard or criterion standard test?

In medical statistics gold standard test usually refers to a diagnostic test or benchmark that is the best available under reasonable conditions
A hypothetical ideal "gold standard" test has a sensitivity of 100% with respect to the presence of the disease (it identifies all individuals with a well defined disease process; it does not have any false-negative results) and a specificity of 100% (it does not falsely identify someone with a condition that does not have the condition; it does not have any false-positive results). In practice, there are sometimes no true "gold standard" tests.

2.3.2 | Teaching

What types of teaching do you know?

1 to 1 teaching
Pros: catered to the individual student, allows gaps in knowledge to be identified and maximizes participation and interaction
Cons: time consuming, heavily relies on teacher-student rapport, can be intimidating, teaching can be too paternalistic, no learning from peers.

Small-Group teaching
Pros: encourages communication and team building, facilitates problem-based learning, teacher acts as mentor guiding group discussion before ideas are shared as small groups come together at the end, students learn from each other.
Cons: some group members can take over discussion, dependent on participation, requires a set pre-course knowledge level of topic.

Didactic Lectures
Pros: Can reach a large audience, can be interactive if pushed,
Cons: not catered to individuals, does not require participation, relies on presenter and slides

E-learning
Pros: can reach large number, allow learners to learn in their own time and promotes self-directed learning, allows distance learning
Cons: needs to be well structured and formally assessed to ensure participation, asking questions can be difficult

How would you organise a weekly SpR/SHO teaching session?

This question tests your logical thinking and also your organisational skills.

If you have previously organised a course or event make sure you mention it and reflect on the learning points.

Example

"I have previously organised a conference so I would utilise my experiences from this:

- I would first utilise feedback on the existing teaching, gain insight from my peers and also outline what I would want teaching to provide
- Involve peers who could help – someone to look after finance, someone to organise speaker practicalities such as parking expenses etc.
- I would look at a national curriculum such as ISCP or FRCS curriculum to define objectives that teaching must achieve
- I would involve a senior consultant with a passion for teaching and evidence-based medicine to oversee the course and recommend speakers
- Define a format such as lectures, SGT, journal club or practical workshops
- I would find a suitable time and location for teaching to take place to maximise attendance, this could be centrally located or rotate around local hospitals
- I would budget for refreshments and ensure I get free room and AV hire to minimise costs
- For any simulation or cadaveric materials I would involve industry and acquire appropriate sponsorship
- As not everyone will be able to attend I would also try to make materials available online and institute pre-reading materials such as journal articles or key topics
- Online sign-up
- Ensure regular contact with attendees and speakers
- Gain feedback and improve subsequent sessions"

2.3.3 Topical obstetrics and gynaecology

What do you understand about the changes being made to the Consultant role in O&G?

The Royal College of Obstetricians and Gynaecologists (RCOG) supports the provision of 24 hour on-site consultant led care. Implementation of a Consultant led service is planned, particularly in high risk delivery suites.

The service provision within NHS trusts require that the majority of consultants must be trained in obstetrics and be competent with managing emergency gynaecological services. However, not all obstetricians and gynaecologists of the future will perform specialised gynaecological surgery.

While there is the need for maintaining acute services in both obstetrics and gynaecology, training will also reflect the need for fewer consultants required to deliver advanced general gynaecological surgery.

Appropriate time should be identified, per week, for consultants' supporting professional activities, including teaching, training, clinical governance and continuing professional development.

Do you think it is a good thing to have resident 24 hour Consultant cover?

Below outlines some of the benefits and disadvantages of a 24 hour Consultant on call in O&G.

Benefits

- It is possible that staff will feel better supported, particularly in the assessment of emergency cases such as a shoulder dystocia where timely intervention is critical. Constant presence of an immediately available consultant improves patient safety.
- There are more opportunities for one to one training with junior staff, for example in cardiotocograph interpretation, surgical skills and management /leadership skills.
- There is continued hands on experience for the consultant, preventing them from becoming deskilled.
- There are more opportunities for a registrar to improve and complete their portfolio as their online mandatory assessments often require a consultant to be present.
- The 'Hospital at Night Study' has confirmed that in obstetrics the level of activity is the same throughout the 24 hour period: a good reason to provide the same level of care at night as in the day.

Disadvantages

- Consultants may become unavailable for elective services during the day time leading to overall adverse impact on other services. Consultants may become deskilled in other areas such as elective gynaecology lists. Furthermore patients might lack continuity of care in these clinics.
- Consultants might suffer chronic tiredness with the feeling of general exhaustion. The concept of continual shift and night time work might place an extra burden on the consultant poising future problems with recruitment and retention of staff. Low staff morale will affect patient care.
- Consultants may end up performing inappropriate tasks for their level. This might take learning opportunities away from the registrar leading to a lack of registrar independence.
- Whether permanent Consultant presence objectively improves standards of care is unclear.

References

The Future Role of the Consultant. Setting standards to improve women's health. The Royal College of Obstetricians and Gynaecologists 2005.
Experiences of a 24 hour resident consultant service. Views and Counter views. Simon Edmonds and Keith Allenby 2008.

What do you understand about the training MATRIX?

The training MATRIX outlines the annual expectation of educational progress from ST1-ST7 in obstetrics and gynaecology. Trainees are assessed against this MATRIX at their ARCPs. If a trainee achieves all of the standards outlined in the MATRIX for that training year, they should be issued with an ARCP outcome 1 (indicating successful transition to the next training year). The matrix defines the minimum standard required and trainees are encouraged to exceed these requirements.

Tell me what standards are expected to be achieved at ST1 level according to the MATRIX?

Below is a summary of the training MATRIX outlined for the ST1 year. Try to familiarise yourself with the headings and expectations.

Standard	Requirement
Progress achieving basic competencies in the e-portfolio log book	The online logbook consists of core training modules 1-19. Progress with these are needed at ST1 level.
Clinical skills	Acting as 1st On call
Formative Objective Structured Assessment of Technical Skills (OSATS)	Fetal blood sampling Manual removal of placenta Uncomplicated caesarean section Non-rotational assisted vaginal delivery (ventouse) Non-rotational assisted vaginal delivery (forceps) Surgical management of miscarriage
At least 3 summative OSATS confirming competence by more than one Consultant. (can be achieved prior to the specified year). Evidence of at least one consultant observed summative OSAT for each item confirming continuing competency since last ARCP	Perineal Repair Opening and closing the abdomen
Mini-Cex -Structured assessment of an observed clinical encounter	8
Case Based Discussions	8
Reflective practice	8
Regional Teaching	Attendance at regional teaching

PORTFOLIO

Standard	Requirement
Obligatory Courses	Basic Practical Skills in Obstetrics and Gynaecology CTG training (usually eLearning package) and other local mandatory training Obstetric simulation course (e.g. PROMPT/ ALSO/other)
Team Observation forms	TO1s at least twice per year without concerns
Clinical governance (patient safety, audit, risk management and quality improvement)	1 completed and presented project Evidence of attendance at local risk management meetings
Teaching Experience	Documented evidence of teaching (e.g. to medical students/ foundation trainees/GPSTs)
Leadership and management experience	Evidence of department responsibility
Presentations and publications (etc)	Department presentation
Trainee Evaluation Form (TEF)	TEF completed on ePortfolio

3 CLINICAL

CLINICAL

3.1 | Asthma

Scenario

A 20-year-old lady who is 34 weeks pregnant presents to the emergency department with acute shortness of breath and wheeze. She admits to not having used her prescribed inhalers for some months but tried her salbutamol, with limited effect, prior to attending. You are called to assess her. On arrival, she is afebrile, tachypnoeic, tachycardic at 105bpm and speaking in partial sentences with saturations of 93%.

What is your differential diagnosis?

- Acute Asthma
- Pulmonary Embolus
- Pneumonia
- Pneumothorax

The most likely diagnosis in this woman is an acute exacerbation of asthma. She has already alluded to inhaler use and presents with acute deterioration featuring wheeze and dyspnoea. Asthma is the most common respiratory pathology encountered in pregnancy, with deterioration occurring most frequently 24 to 36 weeks.

How would you acutely manage this patient?

This patient should be managed with a structured ABCDE approach, with special consideration given to her respiratory and circulatory systems.

Airway: Assess for features of obstruction (stridor/agonal breathing). Her capacity to speak in full sentences allows us to gauge the severity of a potential asthma exacerbation.

Breathing: Supply the patient with high-flow oxygen via a non-rebreathe mask aiming for saturations 94-98%. Her respiratory rate, effort and use of any accessory muscles needs to be assessed. Tracheal position should be palpated to exclude any features of tension pneumothorax. Her lung fields should be percussed and auscultated for any added sounds or reduced air entry. We have been informed that this patient is tachypnoeic with audible wheeze and has a history of inhaler use. It would therefore be appropriate to commence nebulised beta-agonist salbutamol 2.5mg and anti-muscarinic ipratropium bromide 500mcg. These can run continuously in the first instance to aid with her respiratory effort. Oral (Prednisolone) or intravenous (Hydrocortisone) steroid therapy should be administered.

Circulation: Heart rate and rhythm, blood pressure and capillary refill time should be acquired. The patient is tachycardic and insertion of a large bore cannula is required with appropriate bloods drawn (FBC, U+E, LFTs, CRP). Fluid challenges can be considered should she become hypotensive.

Disability: Assess neurological status with either AVPU or GCS systems. Check her blood glucose.

Exposure: Examine the abdomen and check fetal heart rate. Her calves should be assessed for clinical signs of DVT (swelling, tenderness, erythema) and any oedema noted.

What investigations would aid your diagnosis

Peak expiratory flow rate (PEFR) with a result <50% predicted indicative of a severe asthma attack.
Arterial blood gas (ABG) to assess the degree of hypoxia and any element of normal/raised $PaCO_2$
ECG to determine heart rate and rhythm, a sinus tachycardia would be in keeping with her current condition.
Fetal heart rate with Doppler to assess any impact on the fetus.
Continuous fetal monitoring (CTG) is recommended for acute severe asthma exacerbations in pregnancy.
Chest radiograph (CXR) can be considered, although it is not routine unless a life-threatening exacerbation or pneumothorax is suspected.

How would you proceed if there was no response with initial nebuliser therapy and steroids?

Current guidance from the British Thoracic Society (BTS) suggests a step-wise approach to management of acute asthma exacerbations. If response to initial therapy has been poor, then involvement of senior colleagues, including intensive care or respiratory high dependency units should be sought prior to continuation of further therapy:

- Consideration of IV Magnesium Sulphate *(1.2-2g)* if no response to initial treatment
- IV aminophylline *(No significant association of adverse perinatal outcome with PO or IV therapy)*
- Admission to a high dependency or critical care environment for consideration of non-invasive or invasive ventilation

The patient is concerned regarding the effects of using her prescribed maintenance inhalers during pregnancy and has avoided them. How would you counsel her and what would be your advice?

There are two components to this question. First, in order to counsel her effectively:
- Locate a safe and private environment
- Explore and listen to her concerns
- Explain, educate and address concerns in a professional manner, without medical jargon
- Check understanding and clarify any further questions

CLINICAL

- Provide written information and support for out-of-hospital contact and ensure primary care follow-up

What are some of the clinical features of a 'life-threatening' asthma exacerbation?

A life threatening exacerbation is defined as any one of the following clinical signs or measurements in a patient with severe asthma:

	Life Threatening Asthma	
Severe Asthma + **(any one of)**	**Clinical Signs**	**Measurements**
PEFR 33-50% predicted Respiratory rate >25/min Heart rate >110bpm Inability to complete sentences	Altered conscious level Exhaustion Arrhythmia Hypotension Cyanosis Silent chest/poor respiratory effort	PEF <33% SpO2 <92% PaO2 <8kPa "normal" PaCO2 (4-6kPa)

Should this patient be admitted for further monitoring?

The criteria for admission should include any feature of severe or life threatening asthma exacerbation and those whose PEFR is <75% post treatment. The British Thoracic Society suggests that pregnancy is a criterion for admission and further monitoring prior to discharge. In this case the patient is 34 weeks pregnant and has features of a severe asthma attack, therefore admission would be recommended. Once discharged from hospital, primary care follow-up is essential.

What are the risks of poorly-controlled asthma in pregnancy?

Uncontrolled asthma in pregnancy has many associations with maternal and fetal complications including:

- Hyperemesis
- Hypertension/Pre-eclampsia
- Vaginal haemorrhage
- Complicated labour
- Fetal growth restriction
- Premature labour

SUMMARY

Asthma is the most common respiratory disease affecting pregnancy, with up to 18% of sufferers having at least one emergency admission for exacerbation. Evidence exists to show that up to one-third of pregnancies see a deterioration in asthma and this is commonly in those with poorly-controlled disease around conception. The aim of managing chronic asthma in pregnancy focuses on continuation of established maintenance therapy such as inhaled beta-agonists and steroids. The current literature has not established any increased risk in maternal or fetal complications with these therapies.

Acute exacerbations of asthma in pregnancy should be managed in a similar manner to the general population; with use of controlled oxygen, inhaled or nebulised beta-agonists and steroids. The additional consideration of fetal monitoring via doppler or CTG should be considered. The aetiology of exacerbations is multi-factorial, but evidence has suggested that viral respiratory tract infections play an important role and that antibiotics are generally over-prescribed. Escalation to IV aminophylline, salbutamol or the use of non-invasive ventilation should always be managed in a critical care setting following discussion with seniors.

TOP TIPS

➕ Call for senior help early: patients can deteriorate quickly despite adequate initiation of treatment. Make your senior colleagues aware in a timely manner and note that previous intensive care admission for asthma requires referral.

➕ Explore her concerns for not taking her regular inhalers: the clue is in the history where it states she has not been taking her regular inhalers. Exploration of this may pick up further marks and demonstrate your ability to communicate effectively with your patient and your knowledge of the medication advised during pregnancy.

➕ Be mindful of PE as a differential: as with any shortness of breath in pregnancy, you always have to consider VTE given its four-fold increased risk compared to the general population.

CLINICAL

References:
British Thoracic Society and Scottish Intercollegiate Guidelines Network. British Guideline on the Management of Asthma- A national clinical guideline. Revised June 2009.
Greentop Guidelines No 37a. Thrombosis and Embolism during Pregnancy and the Puerperium, Reducing the Risk. Revised 2009.

3.2 | Anaphylaxis

Scenario

A 29-year-old lady is prescribed Benzylpenicillin IV in labour due to her Group B Strep positive status. Shortly after administration by her midwife she develops intense itching, a rash and shortness of breath.

What is your differential diagnosis?

Anaphylactic reaction
Severe asthma attack
Faint (vasovagal episode)
Panic attack
Idiopathic non-allergic urticarial or angio-oedema

How would you acutely manage this patient?

The management of anaphylaxis in pregnancy is largely the same as in the non-pregnant patient.
Call for help
Stop IV infusion

Airway: Look for the signs of airway obstruction. Consider chin tilt and lift, jaw thrust. Consider insertion of an oropharyngeal or nasopharyngeal airway. Anaphylaxis can cause pharyngeal or laryngeal oedema. Overcoming this obstruction may be very difficult and early tracheal intubation is often required. This requires expert help. Give oxygen at high concentration: >10L/min through reservoir mask. Aim sats 94-98%.

Breathing: Look, listen and feel for the general signs of respiratory distress: sweating, central cyanosis, use of the accessory muscles of respiration and abdominal breathing. Assess respiratory rate. A high, or increasing, respiratory rate is a marker of illness and a warning that the patient may deteriorate suddenly. If the patient has stopped breathing, use a pocket mask or two person bag-mask ventilation while calling urgently for expert help. Early tracheal intubation should be considered by someone experienced.

Circulation: Measure HR, BP, CRT. Commence IV Fluid challenge. Large volumes of fluid leak from circulation in anaphylactic reaction. There will also be vasodilation, low blood pressure and signs of shock. Tilt patient onto left lateral position to relieve aortocaval compression. Manual displacement of gravid uterus may be necessary. Insert 2 large bore cannulae. Maintain a systolic BP of above 90mm Hg to ensure adequate placental perfusion. Commence continuous electronic monitoring. CPR and emergency C-section should be performed if indicated.

Disability: Assess conscious level with AVPU or GCS scoring systems. Examine pupils. Check blood glucose to exclude hypoglycaemia.

Exposure: To examine the patient properly, full exposure of the body is necessary. Skin and mucosal changes after anaphylaxis can be subtle. Minimise heat loss.

0.5 mg IM (= 500 micrograms = 0.5 mL of 1:1000) adrenaline
Repeat the IM adrenaline dose if there is no improvement in the patient's condition
Further doses can be given at about 5-minute intervals according to the patient's response
Chlorphenamine 10mg IM or slow IV
Hydrocortisone 200mg IM or slow IV
If history of asthma consider bronchodilators

What investigations would aid your diagnosis

Anaphylaxis is a clinical diagnosis
Bloods for mast cell tryptase – to confirm anaphylaxis. Ideally 3x timed samples at time of reaction, 1-2 hours and 24 hours
ABG to assess oxygenation and lactate
ECG
Continuous fetal monitoring

Why is it necessary to consider early intubation in anaphylaxis?

In an anaphylactic reaction, upper airway obstruction or bronchospasm may make bag mask ventilation difficult or impossible. Laryngeal/pharyngeal oedema and bronchospasm can make early intubation necessary to overcome obstruction.

What common drugs can precipitate anaphylactic reaction?
- Antibiotics
- Opioids
- Non-steroidal anti-inflammatory drugs *(NSAIDs)*
- Intravenous *(IV)* contrast media
- Muscle relaxants
- Other anaesthetic drugs

What symptoms may a patient describe which suggest impending anaphylactic reaction?
- New rash and swelling
- Palpitations and tachycardia
- Nausea, vomiting and abdominal pain
- Feeling faint - with a sense of impending doom
- Intense vulvar and vaginal itching
- Low back pain, uterine cramps, fetal distress
- Preterm labor
- Itching of the palate or external auditory meatus

CLINICAL

- Dyspnoea
- Stridor and wheezing
- Airway swelling, stridor, breathing difficulty, wheeze, cyanosis, hypotension, tachycardia and reduced capillary filling suggest impending severe reaction

What is the risk for the fetus in anaphylactic shock?

The fetus compensates for decreased blood flow by means of redistribution of blood to vital organs, including the brain, heart, placenta, and adrenal glands; increased oxygen uptake and tissue oxygen extraction; and decreased body movements. The level and duration of fetal hypoxia that exceed these compensatory mechanisms, although not precisely defined in human beings, are affected by fetal reserve and gestational age. When these mechanisms fail, the fetus is at risk of hypoxic-ischemic encephalopathy and permanent central nervous system damage, which occur more commonly in the infant than in the mother, and of death, which can occur despite maternal survival.

What are the RCOG guidelines for offering GBS specific intra-partum antibiotics

- Previous baby with invasive GBS infection
- GBS bacteriuria in the current pregnancy
- Vaginal swab positive for GBS in current pregnancy
- Pyrexia *(>38°C)* in labour *(give broad-spectrum antibiotics to include GBS cover)*
- Chorioamnionitis *(give broad-spectrum antibiotics to include GBS cover)*

What is RCOG recommended antibiotic regimen in GBS?

- For women who have accepted IAP, benzylpenicillin should be administered as soon as possible after the onset of labour and given regularly until delivery
- Clindamycin should be administered to those women allergic to benzylpenicillin

How should infants at risk of early onset GBS be managed?

Well infants at risk of EOGBS should be observed for the first 12–24 hours after birth with regular assessments of general wellbeing, feeding, heart rate, respiratory rate and temperature. Postnatal antibiotic prophylaxis is not recommended for asymptomatic term infants without known antenatal risk factors.

SUMMARY

Anaphylaxis in pregnancy is managed as per the non-pregnant patient. Effectiveness of treatment relies on prompt diagnosis and adrenaline administration. It is essential women are positioned on their left side to prevent aortocaval compression. Commence continuous fetal monitoring. Airway complications are common in anaphylaxis and senior anaesthetic support is of upmost importance as early intubation due to largyngeal oedema can be required.

TOP TIPS

➕ The treatment of anaphylactic shock is 0.5 mg IM *(= 500 micrograms = 0.5 mL of 1:1000)* adrenaline

➕ Repeat the IM adrenaline dose if there is no improvement in the patient's condition.

➕ Beware of the patient with concurrent asthma and consider bronchodilators as additional therapy.

➕ Position the patient on left lateral side.

References
Anaphylaxis during pregnancy. Simons, F. Estelle R. et al. Journal of Allergy and Clinical Immunology , Volume 130 , Issue 3 , 597 - 606

CLINICAL

3.3 Early Pregnancy Bleeding

Scenario

A 24-year-old P0 is referred by her GP to the early pregnancy unit with vaginal bleeding and crampy, central abdominal pain. She is 8 weeks pregnant. She is previously fit and well, with no past medical history of note. She feels generally well apart from the pain and bleeding, but very anxious about losing the baby. Observations show a mild tachycardia, but all else are stable. You have been asked to review her.

What is your differential diagnosis?

- Miscarriage
- Ectopic pregnancy
- Molar pregnancy
- Cervical ectropion
- Cervical pathology
- Consider placental position *(accreta or praevia in later pregnancy)*

How would you acutely manage this patient?

An ABCDE approach should be used initially to assess this patient. This should be followed by a detailed history and examination, including speculum examination.

Airway: Assess for evidence of airway obstruction; stridor, abnormal noises. Ensure the patient is able to talk comfortably.

Breathing: Check the oxygen saturations and respiratory rate of the patient. Auscultate all areas of the chest and if concerned commence high flow oxygen (15L via a non re-breathe mask).

Circulation: Assess the heart rate, blood pressure and capillary refill time. Gain IV access (2x large bore cannulae in ante-cubital fossae if bleeding heavily) and take bloods including full blood count, group and save (+/- crossmatch depending on how heavily the patient is bleeding), clotting, beta HCG, renal function and venous blood gas (VBG). VBG gives a quick assessment of Hb, and also overall indicators for how acutely unwell the patient is e.g. lactate, pH. If tachycardia persists, commence IV fluids – 500ml Hartmann's STAT and reassess. Palpate the abdomen, if it is tense and the patient shows signs of peritonism, reconsider diagnoses; is this a ruptured ectopic? If heavy bleeding persists, insert a urinary catheter and monitor urine output with a urometer.

Disability: Assess the consciousness of the patient with AVPU or GCS.

Exposure: Assess temperature, check for any other bleeding sites. Assess how heavily the patient is bleeding by undertaking a speculum examination and observing the cervical os. If pregnancy products are visible in the os, remove them if possible.

What investigations would aid your diagnosis

Urine sample: urine pregnancy test should be tested.
Serum HCG: this confirms pregnancy and is important for follow up.
Rhesus group: this is important to remember in women who are bleeding and pregnant. She may require anti-D if she is Rhesus negative.
TV/TA USS: this will confirm the location of the pregnancy. It can also date the pregnancy accurately and, depending on dates, confirm viability of the pregnancy and presence/absence of a fetal heartbeat (FH). Most USS departments use a BHCG level between 1000-2000 as the level by which a gestational sac should be visible.

How do we classify miscarriage?

- Threatened miscarriage: bleeding +/- pain in an ongoing pregnancy confirmed with bloods *(HCG)* and USS.
- Incomplete miscarriage: the miscarriage has started and pregnancy is not viable. Part of the pregnancy tissue remains in the womb.
- Complete miscarriage: All pregnancy tissue has been passed and the womb is confirmed empty *(be sure to check there is no extra-uterine pregnancy in this case)*.
- Missed/delayed miscarriage: diagnosed on USS, the pregnancy has stopped growing and there is no FH but it remains in the uterus.

How would you manage a threatened miscarriage with confirmed intra-uterine pregnancy and FH on USS?

Explain to the woman that if the bleeding settles/stops she should be reassured and continue the pregnancy as planned.
If bleeding increases or persists after 14 days she should be re-assessed and give her contact details.

What are the management options for miscarriage? How would you decide which to use and what would you counsel about for each?

Expectant, Medical or Surgical. Women should be provided with verbal and written information and allowed to make an informed choice about how to proceed.

Expectant: Use first line for 7-14 days in women diagnosed with miscarriage unless they have a strong preference for alternative method. Not advised if:

- Increased risk of heavy bleeding *(e.g towards end of first trimester, coagulopathies)*
- Previous adverse/traumatic event associated with pregnancy *(e.g. stillbirth, antepartum haemorrhage)*
- Evidence of infection

Explain that most women will pass pregnancy tissue spontaneously and warn about pain/expected heaviness of bleeding. Provide/advise where to get adequate pain relief from and provide written information about what to expect and emergency advice.

If bleeding and pain settle in 7-14 days, advise to take urine pregnancy test in 3 weeks and to return if still positive.

Advise that if expectant management does not work (bleeding does not occur or persists beyond 14 days) she may need a repeat scan and medical/surgical management.

Medical: 800 microgram of misoprostol orally or vaginally depending on the woman's preference. Explain side effects (pain, vomiting diarrhoea).

Advise her if bleeding has not started in 24 hours to contact as she may need a further dose of misoprostol. If still not successful she may require surgical management.

Provide adequate analgesia and anti-emetics – in hospital or at home.

Explain what is expected and provide written information about the process and emergency advice.

Advise her to check a urine pregnancy test 3 weeks later and if still positive to contact department.

Surgical: If clinically appropriate offer a choice of manual vacuum aspiration under local anaesthetic in a clinic/outpatient setting, or surgical management in theatre under general anaesthetic.

Discuss risks procedure: bleeding, infection, perforation of uterus, damage to surrounding structures: bladder, ureters, bowel and blood vessels, risk of venous thromboembolism.

What would you advise about future pregnancies?

Allow time to come to terms with this miscarriage and grieve. Miscarriages are common and most are sporadic. There is nothing she could have done to prevent it and most occur because of chromosomal abnormalities and the baby would not survive. There is a good chance she will have a normal pregnancy in the future.

When would we expect to see a FH on TV USS? What would you do if you could not identify it?

When the cord-rump-length (CRL) of the fetal pole is >7mm. If <7mm, rescan in 7-10 days to reassess growth and presence of FH. Remember not to rely on LMP to date the pregnancy and explain this to the patient. If CRL >7mm and no FH identified, confirm this with another technician and re-scan in 7-10 days to assess for growth and confirm miscarriage.

What would you do if you could not see a fetal pole on TV USS?

Measure the mean sac diameter (MSD) of the gestation sac: if it is <25mm then rescan in 7-10 days. If greater than 25 mm, seek a second opinion to try and confirm the diagnosis of miscarriage, and rescan in 7-10 days to confirm no change.

SUMMARY

Bleeding in early pregnancy is a common presentation and many patients continue to have a normal pregnancy with no ongoing complications. It is a distressing time for patients and must be dealt with sensitively. It is important to provide clear advice, including safety netting and good written information wherever possible. Encourage patients to make an informed choice of management options for miscarriage unless clinically indicated. It is important not to forget the psychological sequelae of miscarriage, and to provide information on support and counselling services available. If repeated miscarriage, make appropriate referrals to recurrent miscarriage or other available clinics.

TOP TIPS

➕ Never forget to exclude an ectopic pregnancy in any woman of child bearing age presenting with bleeding +/- pain!

➕ Make sure you show off your excellent communications skills in a situation like this – allow the patient time to speak, ask about concerns and questions and offer small chunks of information at a time. They probably won't take everything in at once and may not need a lot of technical information. Remember to offer written information; it is particularly useful when breaking bad news.

➕ Don't forget to stress safety advice if patients are going home. Clear advice about what they should expect and what to watch out for, when to seek help and who/where to get it from, phone numbers etc.

CLINICAL

References:
Ectopic Pregnancy and Miscarriage: diagnosis and initial management. NICE guidelines [CG154], Dec 2012
Bleeding and Pain in Early Pregnancy: information for you. Royal college of Obstetrics & Gynaecology. Jan 2008

3.4 Leg Swelling

Scenario

A 67-year-old woman has presented to the emergency department with a swollen left lower leg. The swelling was an acute onset overnight and is associated with pain, erythema and throbbing. She recently under went surgery for an endometrial malignancy, she recalls this as a hysterectomy. Her BMI is 24 and she is clinically well. You have been asked to review to her.

What is your differential diagnosis?

Deep vein thrombosis (DVT)
Lymphoedema
Thrombophlebitis
Peripheral oedma, heart failure, cirrhosis, nephrotic syndrome.
Cellulitis
Gout
Compartment syndrome
Musculoskeletal
Trauma

The likely answer is a DVT and this should be top of your differentials. She has two risk factors including being post surgical and having a malignancy.
During your assessment it is important to assess both legs as many of the other differential diagnosis would present bilaterally.
Question the patient of her gynaecological procedure and her condition before discharge. Many patients are sent home on anticoagulation however do not take it. It is uncommon for someone on prophylactic anticoagulation if taken appropriately to suffer a DVT. Make sure you ask her about this.

How would you acutely manage this patient?

Airway: Assess the patient's ability to talk in full sentences.

Breathing: Respiratory rate and oxygen saturations. Auscultate lung fields.

Circulation: Assess blood pressure, capillary refill time, heart rate and rhythm. Draw off bloods including FBC, U+E, LFTs CRP, D-dimer. Examine for circulatory features of cynanosis in the leg/foot.

Disability: Examine conscious level using AVPU or GCS scoring system.

Exposure: Examine for other signs that might identify the source of this swelling. Measure the legs.
Calculate a DVT probability score eg Wells' Score.

What investigations would aid your diagnosis

Baseline bloods should be taken before taking anticoagulant therapy. Blood should be taken for a full blood count, coagulation screen, urea and electrolytes, liver function tests and a bone profile.
D-dimer
Duplex USS
If clinical suspicion high but investigations inconclusive consider venography, CT or MRI.

What are the factors that increase the risk of thrombosis post operatively?

- Malignancy
- Age >60
- Smoking
- Obesity *(BMI >30kg/m2)*
- Thrombotic disorders *(eg Factor V Leiden)*
- Previous thrombosis
- Family history of thrombosis
- Immobilisation period
- Comorbidities *(heart failure)*
- Varicose veins
- Dehydration

What are the other potential presenting features?

- Limb pain & tenderness along the line of the deep veins
- Swelling of the calf/thigh usually unilateral
- Pitting oedema
- Distension of the superficial veins
- Increase in skin temperature
- Skin discolouration

Describe a diagnostic scoring system for DVTs

Wells diagnostic algorithm
Because of the unreliability of clinical features, diagnostic scoring systems have been validated to classify patients as having a high, intermediate or low probability of developing DVT, based on history and clinical examination.

Score one point for each of the following:

- Active cancer *(treatment ongoing or within the previous six months, or palliative)*
- Paralysis, paresis or recent plaster immobilisation of the legs
- Recently bedridden for three days or more, or major surgery within the previous 12 weeks, requiring general or regional anaesthesia

CLINICAL

- Localised tenderness along the distribution of the deep venous system *(such as the back of the calf)*
- Entire leg is swollen
- Calf swelling by more than 3 cm compared with the asymptomatic leg *(measured 10 cm below the tibial tuberosity)*
- Pitting oedema confined to the symptomatic leg
- Collateral superficial veins *(non-varicose)*
- Previously documented DVT

Subtract two points if an alternative cause is considered at least as likely as DVT.

The risk of DVT is likely if the score is two or more, and unlikely if the score is one or less.

SUMMARY

Thrombotic events post operatively are becoming less common due to active prophylaxis regimes. It is important to take all patients seriously when they present. Treatment should be commenced as soon as possible and not delayed while awaiting definitive investigation. For oncology patients the way in which the procedure was performed is also important. Robotic cases are being performed more frequently and rare complications such as compartment syndrome are occurring. It is important that their gynaecology and oncology team are made aware the diagnosis as it may affect further treatment planning.

TOP TIPS

➕ Always treat a suspected DVT until its proven its not I.E. while awaiting investigation.

➕ If a patient presents with a DVT and no cause found then <40 think thrombophilia, over 40 think cancer.

➕ If malignancy present then treatment is required for 6 months *(i.e. longer.)*

References:
Watson L, Broderick C, Armon MP; Thrombolysis for acute deep vein thrombosis. Cochrane Database Syst Rev. 2014 Jan
Venous thromboembolic diseases: the management of venous thromboembolic diseases and the role of thrombophilia testing; NICE Clinical Guideline. 2012 June

3.5 | Seizure

Scenario

You are an ST1 and fast bleeped to A&E to review a patient at 34 weeks gestation with a BP of 196/115. When you arrive she is having what appears to be a tonic-clonic seizure.

What is your differential diagnosis?

Eclampsia
Primary generalised epilepsy
Hypoglycaemia
Amniotic fluid embolism
Central venous sinus thrombosis
Phaeochromocytoma
Local anaesthetic toxicity e.g. epidural
Overdose e.g. tricyclic antidepressants

How would you acutely manage this patient?

Call for help

Airway: Place the patient in the recovery position if possible to minimize risk of airway compromise. Consider head tilt, chin lift and jaw thrust. If the airway still appears compromised insert an oropharyngeal airway. Use suction to clear airway secretions. Contact the on call anaesthetist as soon as possible.

Breathing: Give high flow O2 (15L via non-rebreathe mask). Assess respiratory rate, oxygen saturations and air entry.

Circulation: Assess BP, capillary refill time and pulse. Insert 2x large bore cannulae.

Disability: Assess conscious level using GCS or AVPU. MgSO4 is the drug of choice to control eclamptic seizures.
Loading dose: magnesium sulphate 4g IV over 20 minutes.
Maintenance dose: magnesium sulphate IV 1 g per hour.
Recurrent seizures whilst on magnesium sulphate: Further bolus of MgSO4 2g IV over 5 minutes. If possible take blood for magnesium levels before bolus. Consider using other forms of medication including general anaesthesia.

Exposure: Examine for other causes of seizure including CVS, RS, abdomen (assess fetal condition with CTG), neuro including reflexes, pupils and examine for papilloedema.

Once patient stabilised, senior decision is required to expedite delivery.

CLINICAL

What investigation would aid your diagnosis

ABG: To assess oxygenation, pH and lactate. Acidosis, poor oxygenation and/or high lactate may demonstrate need for urgent critical care input
FBC: To assess platelet count
LFT's: To assess for HELLP syndrome
U&E's: deranged electrolytes as cause of seizure e.g. hypercalcaemia. Also to assess end organ damage for severe PET
Clotting: To assess for DIC
Urinary PCR
Toxicology screen / Anticonvulsant drug levels (if indicated)
Blood glucose: To check hypoglycaemia not cause
Catheterise: Urometer
Continuous fetal monitoring
Consider CT Head once seizures controlled

What are some risk factors for pre-eclampsia?

Nulliparity
Age > 40
Last pregnancy >10 years ago
Obesity
Family history of pre-eclampsia
Multiple pregnancy
Essential hypertension
Previous history of PET
Chronic kidney disease
Diabetes
Autoimmune disease e.g. SLE

What are some indicators of severe PET?

Systolic BP>160mmHg
Diastolic BP>110mmHg
Proteinuria +++ or PCR >30
Raised serum creatinine >100
Platelets <100
Increased AST or ALT
Epigastric pain
Headache, other cerebral or visual symptoms
Retinal haemorrhages or papilloedema
Pulmonary oedema

What is the definition of eclampsia?

Seizures occurring in pregnancy or within 10 days of delivery and with at least two of the following features documented within 24 hours of the seizure:

- Hypertension diastolic blood pressure *(DBP)* of at least 90 mm Hg *(if DBP less than 90 mm Hg on booking visit)* or DBP increment of 25 mm Hg above booking level.
- Proteinuria one *"**plus**"* or at least 0.3 g/24 h.

- Thrombocytopenia less than 100 000/µl.
- Raised aspartate amino transferase *(AST)* greater than 42 IU/l.

What monitoring would you request for a patient on MgSO4?

Magnesium toxicity causes loss of tendon reflexes, followed by respiratory depression and ultimately, respiratory arrest. Toxic levels are unlikely to be reached with a maintenance dose of 1 g per hour and a good urine output.

- Deep tendon reflexes hourly *(biceps tendon if epidural in situ)*
- Hourly urine measurements
- Continuous pulse oximetry

Oxygen saturation < 95% in air should raise concern regarding Mg toxicity or pulmonary oedema.

Once seizures have been controlled, what drugs are used to control blood pressure?

First line is labetalol. If the woman can tolerate oral therapy, an initial 200mg oral dose can be given. This can be done before IV access is obtained and so can achieve as quick a result as an initial intravenous dose. A second oral dose can be given after 30 minutes if needed.

If no response or oral therapy not tolerated, repeated boluses of labetalol 50mg followed by a labetalol infusion.

Contraindication: severe asthma, use with caution in women with pre-existing cardiac disease. Second choice agents include hydralazine and nifedipine.

What proportion of seizures occur antepartum, intrapartum and postpartum?

Up to 38% of cases of eclampsia can occur without premonitory signs or symptoms of pre-eclampsia, that is, hypertension, proteinuria, and oedema. Only 38% of eclamptic seizures occur antepartum; 18% occur during labour and a further 44% occur postpartum. Rare cases of eclampsia have occurred over a week after delivery.

What are some of the possible poor outcomes for eclampsia?

Outcome is poor for mother and child. Almost one in 50 women suffering eclamptic seizures die, 23% will require ventilation and 35% will have at least one major complication including pulmonary oedema, renal failure, disseminated intravascular coagulation, HELLP syndrome, acute respiratory distress syndrome, stroke, or cardiac arrest. Stillbirth or neonatal death occurs in approximately one in 14 cases of eclampsia.

What are the aims of postpartum fluid management in severe PET?

Women are at high risk of fluid overload and severe pulmonary oedema. Following delivery, the woman should be fluid restricted in order to wait for the natural diuresis which usually occurs sometime around 36-48 hours post delivery. The total amount of fluid (the total of intravenous and oral fluids) should be restricted

CLINICAL

to 80 ml/hour. Restriction will usually be continued for the duration of magnesium sulphate treatment; however, increased fluid intake may be allowed by a consultant obstetrician at an earlier time point in the presence of significant diuresis.

SUMMARY

Eclamptic seizures require multidisciplinary specialist input to manage effectively. Management focuses around ABCDE approach. It is important to consider other common causes of seizure as listed above. Prompt MgSo4 administration and control of blood pressure with Labetalol or second line agents. If pregnant, it is crucial to expedite delivery once patient is stable. Patients need regular monitoring of bloods (FBC, LFTs, clotting), reflexes, urine output and oxygen saturations. Outcomes can be poor for mother and baby post eclamptic seizure as are high risk for pulmonary oedema, renal failure, stroke, DIC, HELLP syndrome, ARDS and stillbirth.

TOP TIPS

➕ Feel confident in describing the processes for airway management as this can often become occluded in prolonged seizure and is a first priority to stabilise.

➕ Recalling the doses of bolus and maintenance MgSO4 will make you appear slick and knowledgeable.

➕ Most eclamptic seizures happen postpartum.

References:
Douglas KA, Redman CWG. Eclampsia in the United Kingdom. BMJ1994;309:1395–400.

3.6 | Acute Pelvic Pain (1)

Scenario

A 28-year-old woman was admitted to A&E with pelvic pain. She has previously been treated for pelvic inflammatory disease and her last menstrual period was 6 weeks ago. On examination she is very tender in the right iliac fossa. She is tachycardic and hypotensive. You are asked to review her.

What is your differential diagnosis?

- Ectopic pregnancy
- Appendicitis
- Salpingitis
- Ruptured corpus luteum cyst or ovarian follicle
- Spontaneous abortion or threatened abortion
- Ovarian torsion
- Urinary tract Infection

How would you acutely manage this patient?

As for any acute admission, this patient should have a full ABCDE assessment and stabilised before a detailed history is taken.

Airway: Examine for signs of a compromised airway.

Breathing: This should be assessed with saturations, respiratory rate, and auscultation of her chest. As she is acutely unwell high flow oxygen should be administered i.e. 15 litres through a non-rebreathe mask.

Circulation: This includes capillary refill, heart rate and rhythm (with an ECG) and blood pressure. Assessment of her circulation is particularly paramount in this case as she is haemodynamically unstable with hypotension and tachycardia. IV access with two large bore cannulas should be obtained and IV fluid started. Routine bloods including FBC, U+Es, CRP and LFTs with the addition of a serum hCG and cross match should be taken at the time of cannulation. Strict fluid monitoring including measured urine output should be commenced.

Disability: Examine for reduced level of consciousness using GCS scoring system.

Exposure: Examine for any other causes of the patient's tachycardia and hypotension. An abdominal and internal vaginal examination should be performed. She should be commenced on analgesia and kept nil by mouth ahead of a likely operation.

An ectopic pregnancy is highly likely in this case and given her signs of instabil-

CLINICAL

ity she is likely to need urgent surgical intervention. An anaesthetist will need to be contacted urgently for assessment.

What investigations would aid your diagnosis?

Bloods: including FBC, CRP, U+Es, LFTs, venous lactate and cross match. Consider taking blood cultures If the patient has a temperature >38 degrees or signs of sepsis.

Serum hCG and repeat 48 hours later:

- A rise of >66% suggests an intrauterine pregnancy
- Suboptimal rise is suspicious of an ectopic but not diagnostic

Serum progesterone: <20mmol/L highly suggestive of a failing pregnancy.

Urine dip: should be performed to screen for a UTI. If positive send for MC&S.

High vaginal swab

Transvaginal ultrasound scan: to establish the location of the pregnancy, the presence of adnexal mass or free fluid. Identifies an ectopic pregnancy in 90% of cases.

Laparoscopy: gold standard but only indicated when clinically necessary.

What is the incidence of ectopic pregnancy?

The incidence of ectopic pregnancy is 1-2:100 pregnancies. The incidence is increasing.

What are the common examination findings of an ectopic pregnancy?

Common examination findings include:

- Pelvic tenderness
- Adnexal tenderness
- Abdominal tenderness

Other reported signs:

- Cervical motion tenderness
- Brown vaginal discharge
- Rebound tenderness or peritoneal signs
- Shoulder tip pain *(due to haemoperitoneum irritating the diaphragm)*
- Pallor
- Abdominal distension
- Enlarged uterus
- Tachycardia *(more than 100 beats per minute)* or hypotension *(less than 100/60 mmHg)*
- Shock or collapse
- Orthostatic hypotension

What are some of the risk factors for an ectopic pregnancy?

Aged over 40 years old

Smoking
History of pelvic inflammatory disease
Endometriosis
Previous ectopic pregnancy
Previous surgery involving the fallopian tubes (for example sterilisation)
Progesterone only contraception (mini-pill)
In vitro fertilisation or intracytoplasmic sperm injection pregnancy

What are the management options for a patient with an ectopic pregnancy?

Expectant: Expectant management is also suitable for women with an ultrasound diagnosis of an ectopic pregnancy, with minimal symptoms, a decreasing serum hCG that is less than 1000 iU/l at presentation and less than 100 ml of fluid and no evidence of blood in the Pouch of Douglas on ultrasound. These women should be monitored with twice weekly serum hCGs (ideally less than 50% of its initial level within one week) and weekly transvaginal ultrasound examinations.

Medical: This is appropriate management for women with a confirmed (on serum hCG and transvaginal USS) ectopic pregnancy who are clinically well. Women with a serum hCG below 3000 iu/l and minimal symptoms are most suitable.

Medical management is with methotrexate given as a single dose based on body surface area (usual dose between 75 mg and 90mg). Serum hCG levels are checked on days 4 and 7. Further doses are given if the serum hCG level fails to fall by 15% between days 4 and 7. 14% of women require more than one dose. Women should be advised to avoid sexual intercourse during treatment and to use reliable contraception for 3 months as methotrexate is associated with teratogenic risk. 10% medically managed go on to require surgical intervention.

Surgical: Laparoscopy is preferred to laparotomy as it is associated with shorter hospital stays, less blood loss and lower analgesia requirements. If the patient is haemodynamically unstable a laparotomy is more appropriate as it is quicker.

What side effects are experienced with methotrexate?

Side effects of methotrexate therapy include conjunctivitis, stomatitis and gastrointestinal upset. Many women also experience abdominal pain although this is often difficult to distinguish from the pain associated with the ectopic pregnancy itself. All women receiving methotrexate for medical management of an ectopic pregnancy should be counselled in regard to the symptoms experienced with treatment.

What further management should be considered when managing a suspected ectopic pregnancy?

Non-sensitised women who are rhesus negative with a confirmed or suspected ectopic should receive anti-D immunoglobulin.

What are some of the less common sites for an ectopic pregnancy?

Less common sites include cervical, ovarian, caesarean section scars and interstitial pregnancies. There is no universally agreed management for these patients so specialist help should be sought.

SUMMARY

Ectopic pregnancy should be a differential diagnosis in any women of reproductive age presenting with abdominal or pelvic pain. A thorough gynaecological history including sexual history should be taken as well as screening for risk factors for an ectopic pregnancy. Serum hCGs and transvaginal ultrasound scan will confirm the diagnosis in the majority of cases. 98% of ectopics are tubal in nature. However, the clinical presentation of an ectopic pregnancy varies dramatically and atypical presentations are common. A minority present with haemodynamic instability and are a gynaecological emergency. Management can either be expectant, medical or surgical depending on the presentation of the patient.

TOP TIPS

➕ Remember that all women of reproductive age presenting with abdominal pain should be considered pregnant until proven otherwise – they all need a pregnancy test!

➕ There is no evidence that examining these patients increases the risk of developing a ruptured ectopic. It is more important to examine them so you do not miss clinical indications of an ectopic.

References:
Collins S, Arulkumaran S, Hayes K, Jackson S, Impey L. Oxford Handbook of Obstetrics and Gynaecology. 3rd edition. Early pregnancy problems: Ectopic Pregnancy; 2013.

National Institute for Health and Care Excellence. NICE guidelines [CG154]: Ectopic pregnancy and miscarriage: diagnosis and initial management; 2012.

3.7 | Pruritus

Scenario

A 26-year-old woman in her first pregnancy presents at 36 weeks complaining of itching particularly focused to the palms of her hands, resulting in her having trouble sleeping. She does not have a rash. Blood tests have been taken but the results are pending. You have been asked to review her.

What is your differential diagnosis?

Obstetric cholestasis
Dermatographia artefacta
Eczema
Pruritic urticarial papules and plaques of pregnancy
Atopic eruption of pregnancy
Pemphygoid gestationis
Pompholyx dermatitis

Pruitis is common in pregnancy, but most other differentials result in a rash, unlike obstetric cholestasis. For this reason it is important to perform careful clinical examination of all patients paying particular attention to the location and type of rash if present. One must consider if skin markings are as a result of rash or trauma secondary to intense itching.

How would you acutely manage this patient?

Initially this patient should have an ABCD assessment
After this a full obstetric history and patient assessment should be performed in a timely manner

In this history ask about:
Fetal movements
Previous pregnancies, history of obstetric cholestasis (90% recurrence rate)
Enquire about signs of cholestasis such as jaundice, dark urine and pale stools
Previous medical history and family history questioning should include obstetric cholestasis, hepatitis C and gallstones

Full clinical examination:
Inspection of any rashes
Abdominal palpation for fetal presentation and size (symphysis fundal height)
Vital observations
CTG monitoring
Urinalysis

What investigations would aid your diagnosis

Bloods: Bile salts will likely be deranged in obstetric cholestasis, with normal LFTs unless in severe cases (remember a raised ALP in pregnancy is likely of placental origin). FBC and biochemistry to ensure normal.
Urine sample

What is the epidemiology for obstetric cholestasis in the UK?

Obstetric cholestasis is uncommon, affecting approximately 7 in 1000 women in the UK. It is more common in women of Indian-Asian or Pakistani-Asian origin, increasing up to 15 in 1000 women (1.5%).

What is the pathophysiology of this condition?

The cause of obstetric cholestasis is not fully understood but thought to be multifactorial, including hormones and genetic factors. Oestrogen may affect the livers management of bile salts resulting in reduced flow and hence build up in the body. Whilst being more common in certain ethnic groups, obstetric cholestasis has also been found to run in families and recur in subsequent pregnancies.

What alternative diagnoses may result in pruritis and abnormal LFTs and how would you investigate further?

- Hepatitis
- Epstein Barr Virus
- Cytomegalovirus
- Primary Biliary Cirrhosis
- Gallstones
- Pre-eclampsia
- Acute fatty liver of pregnancy

Liver autoimmune screen, viral screen, liver ultrasound scan (liver abnormalities and gallstones)

What additional risk factors are associated with obstetric cholestasis?

Obstetric cholestasis increases the incidence of premature birth and meconium passage – in view of this the patient is considered high risk and therefore should be under consultant led care and delivered on the high risk delivery suite. There is also an increased risk of fetal distress in labour, need for emergency caesarean section and post partum haemorrhage. There is no evidence to suggest an increased risk of stillbirth.

How should this patient be managed in the antenatal setting?

On going management should include weekly general obstetric review to include CTG, blood pressure monitoring, urine dip and LFTs. A coagulation screen should also be performed in view of the livers effect on prothromin time. Some cases would benefit from vitamin K administration, however this would be on an individual basis due to risks including neonatal haemolytic anaemia, hyperbiliru-binaemia and kernicterus.

Describe the treatment for obstetric cholestasis.

Treatment focuses on both symptom relief and safe delivery.

Symptom relief has no relation to evidence based improvement in fetal and neonatal outcomes, however can include topical emollients, antihistamines and ursodeoxycholic acid in the improvement of LFTs and pruritus. Ursodeoxycholic acid works to displace more of the hydrophobic endogenous bile salts from the bile acid pool which is thought to protect hepatocyte membranes from bile salt toxicity, hence enhancing bile acid clearance across the placenta away from the fetus.

Elective delivery is advised at 37 weeks gestation due to increased risk of peri-natal and maternal morbidity beyond this stage, however this may be brought forward, for example, in the case of deranged bloods.

SUMMARY

Obstetric cholestasis is an uncommon multifactorial condition of pregnancy outlined by abnormal liver function tests and pruritis as a result of the build up of bile acids in the body. It is important to rule out other causes of such signs and symptoms. Is it thought that the hormonal effects of oestrogen in addition to genetic and environmental factors are causative, including multiple pregnancies and patients with hepatitis C. Symptoms are best treated using ursodeoxycholic acid and usually resolve after birth. This condition should be managed under consultant led care in view of potential risks and both maternal and fetal morbid-ity. In addition, some case studies have identified data to suggest that obstetric cholestasis is associated with an increased risk of stillbirth.

CLINICAL

TOP TIPS

➕ This is a fairly obvious diagnosis from the outset, however it is ex-tremely important to approach this station in a systematic fashion by focusing on a thorough history in order to demonstrate your knowledge of the condition. In light of this, you will likely score well by enquiring about previous obstetric and family obstetric history.

➕ During the examination, verbalising what you are looking for and what you are ruling out *(rashes, for example)* would also demon-strate a sound understanding of your differential diagnosis.

3.8 Shortness of Breath

Scenario

A 40-year-old multiparous woman has presented to the day assessment unit with shortness of breath at 30 weeks pregnant. It was acute onset associated with palpitations and she feels generally unwell. Her BMI is 37 and she reports to be an ex-smoker.

She is slightly tachycardic with a respiratory rate of 30. You have been asked to review to her.

What is your differential diagnosis?

Pulmonary embolus
Cardiomyopathy
Myocardial Infarction
Asthma
Respiratory tract infection

The most likely answer is a PE. She has some risk factors – BMI/ age/ parity. Thrombosis is one of the most common causes of maternal death and therefore when suspected needs swift assessment/treatment until excluded. These patients are often overlooked. A normal blood gas (or respiratory alkalosis) with tachypnoea is relatively common.

How would you acutely manage this patient?

Airway: Examine for signs of airway obstruction. Assess the patient's ability to talk in full sentences.

Breathing: Check oxygen saturations and auscultate lung fields. Supply the patient with high flow oxygen (15L) via a non-rebreathe mask. High flow oxygen should be administered to all acutely ill patients.

Circulation: Assess blood pressure, capillary refill time, heart rate and rhythm. We have been informed that this patient is tachycardic so it is appropriate to insert a large bore cannula. Whilst inserting the cannula draw off bloods including FBC, U+E, LFTs CRP. Examine for circulatory features of cynanosis. Perform an arterial blood gas.

Disability: Examine conscious level using AVPU or GCS scoring system.

Exposure: Examine for other signs that might identify the source of this patients tachypnoea and tachycardia.

Perform a CTG.
If suspicion for a PE is high swift treatment with an anticoagulant such enoxapa-

rin is required and then move onto further investigations.

What investigations would aid your diagnosis

Baseline bloods: should be taken before starting anticoagulant therapy. A full blood count, coagulation screen, urea and electrolytes and liver function tests.
Arterial Blood Gas: Looking for hypoxia although this tends to be less helpful in pregnancy and doesn't exclude a PE if normal.
ECG: The most common abnormalities are T wave inversion, S1Q3T3 pattern and right bundle branch block.
Chest X-ray (CXR): While it is normal in over half, abnormal features caused by PE include atelectasis, effusion, focal opacities or pulmonary oedema. It may identify other pulmonary disease such as pneumonia, pneumothorax or lobar collapse.
(NOTE: The radiation dose to the fetus from a CXR performed at any stage of pregnancy is negligible).
Imaging: In women with suspected PE without symptoms and signs of DVT, a ventilation/perfusion (V/Q) lung scan or a (CTPA) should be performed. When the chest X-ray is abnormal, CTPA should be performed in preference to a V/Q scan. Women should be advised that, compared with CTPA, V/Q scanning may carry a slightly increased risk of childhood cancer but is associated with a lower risk of maternal breast cancer; in both situations, the absolute risk is very small. Performing a thrombophilia screen prior to therapy is not recommended. D-dimer testing should not be performed in the investigation of acute VTE in pregnancy. Clinicians should be aware that, at present, there is no evidence to support the use of pretest probability assessment in the management of acute VTE in pregnancy.
In women with suspected PE who also have symptoms and signs of DVT, compression duplex ultrasound should be performed. If this confirms the presence of DVT, no further investigation is necessary and treatment for VTE should continue.

What are some risk factors for antenatal thrombosis?

Smoking
Obesity (BMI >30kg/m2)
Multiparity
Thrombotic disorders (eg Factor V Leiden)
Previous thrombosis
Family history of thrombosis
Increasing maternal age (>35)
Immobilisation period
Comorbidities (especially inflammatory conditions eg Inflammatory Bowel Disease)
Varicose veins

What are the other potential presenting features?

DVT: leg pain and discomfort (the left is more commonly affected), swelling, tenderness, oedema, increased temperature and a raised white cell count. There may also be abdominal pain. The difficulty is that some of these symptoms may

CLINICAL

be found in normal pregnancies.

PE: dyspnoea, pleuritic chest pain, haemoptysis, faintness, collapse. The patient may have focal signs in the chest, tachypnoea, a raised jugular venous pressure, and there may be ECG changes. Arterial blood gases taken with the patient sitting down may show respiratory alkalosis and hypoxaemia.

What is the therapeutic dose of LMWH in pregnancy?

LMWH should be given in doses titrated against the woman's booking or early pregnancy weight. There is insufficient evidence to recommend whether the dose of LMWH should be given once daily or in two divided doses. Traditionally it is given as 1mg/kg BD.

Can vitamin K antagonists be used during pregnancy for the maintenance treatment of VTE?

Vitamin K antagonists cross the placenta readily and are associated with a characteristic embryopathy following fetal exposure in the first trimester. Other adverse pregnancy outcomes associated include miscarriage, prematurity, low birthweight, neurodevelopmental problems and fetal and neonatal bleeding. Because of their adverse effects on the fetus, vitamin K antagonists, such as warfarin, should not be used for antenatal VTE treatment.

How should massive life-threatening PE in pregnancy and the puerperium be managed?

Collapsed, shocked women who are pregnant or postnatal should be assessed by a team of experienced clinicians including the on-call consultant obstetrician. Women should be managed on an individual basis: intravenous unfractionated heparin, thrombolytic therapy or thoracotomy and surgical embolectomy. Management should involve a multidisciplinary team including senior physicians, obstetricians and radiologists.

Intravenous unfractionated heparin is the preferred, initial treatment in massive PE with cardiovascular compromise.

The on-call medical team should be contacted immediately. An urgent portable echocardiogram or CTPA within 1 hour of presentation should be arranged.

How should anticoagulation be managed postnatally?

Therapeutic anticoagulant therapy should be continued for the duration of the pregnancy and for at least 6 weeks postnatally and until at least 3 months of treatment has been given in total. Before discontinuing treatment the continuing risk of thrombosis should be assessed.

Women should be offered a choice of LMWH or oral anticoagulant for postnatal therapy after discussion about the need for regular blood tests for monitoring of warfarin, particularly during the first 10 days of treatment.

Postpartum warfarin should be avoided until at least the fifth day and for longer in women at increased risk of postpartum haemorrhage.

Women should be advised that neither heparin (unfractionated or LMWH) nor warfarin is contraindicated in breastfeeding.

What happens after the delivery?

Postnatal review for patients who develop VTE during pregnancy or the puerperium should, whenever possible, be at an obstetric medicine clinic or a joint obstetric haematology clinic. Thrombophilia testing should be performed once anticoagulant therapy has been discontinued only if it is considered that the results would influence the woman's future management (i.e. no other risk factors for thrombosis, family history.)

SUMMARY

Thrombotic events in obstetric patients are becoming increasingly common. It is important to take all patients seriously when they present. Treatment should be commenced as soon as possible and not delayed while awaiting investigation. If the patient is close to their delivery date or early labouring it is vital that imaging is performed with the utmost urgency as anticoagulation effects will complicate the delivery adding extra risk. There are evolving thoughts that antenatal prophylaxis may be required for those patients at high risk (eg morbidly obese) however no guidance exists. The postnatal period needs to be covered with anticoagulation therapy with at least a total of 3 months post event or 6 weeks post delivery whichever is longer.

TOP TIPS

➕ Do not assume a normal ABG excludes a PE in pregnancy.

➕ Always treat a suspected PE until its proven its not one ie. while awaiting investigation.

➕ Always take a family history of thrombosis, and ask about all other risk factors.

➕ Do not forget to counsel women of risks *(all be them low)* of imaging and gain consent prior to requesting.

CLINICAL

References:
Centre for Maternal and Child Enquiries (CMACE). Saving Mothers' Lives: reviewing maternal deaths to make motherhood safer: 2006–08. The Eighth Report on Confidential

Enquiries into Maternal Deaths in the United Kingdom. BJOG 2011;118 Suppl 1:1–203.

Acute management of thrombosis and embolism during pregnancy and the puerperium; Green-top Guideline No 37, February 2007

3.9   Fever and Discharge

Scenario

You are called to review a 20-year-old woman in the emergency department. She feels unwell, with lower abdominal pain and new vaginal discharge for a few days. She has a negative pregnancy test and has a temperature of 38°C and a heart rate of 110bpm.

What is your differential diagnosis?

Pelvic Inflammatory Disease (PID)
Pyelonephritis
Appendicitis
Ovarian cyst accident (rupture, haemorrhage)
Adnexal torsion
Renal colic
Gastroenteritis
Endometriosis
Degenerating fibroid

How would you acutely manage this patient?

Management should begin with an ABCDE approach.

Airway/Breathing: Ensure the airway is protected and assess her breathing for any signs of respiratory distress or chest infection, given she is febrile. Start high flow O2 (15L/min). Note that tachypnoea is an early marker of the unwell patient.

Circulation: Assess her circulation for signs of septic shock e.g. being peripherally cold, and for hypotension. Site a cannula and give intravenous (IV) fluids, especially if she is hypotensive.

Disability: Assess her consciousness using AVPU or the GCS.

Once the patient is stable take a history. Determine the location and character of the pain, in particular if it is bilateral lower abdominal pain, and whether she has dyspareunia. Determine if the vaginal discharge is offensive e.g. noticeable bad smell and if there is a history of abnormal vaginal bleeding e.g. intermenstrual or post-coital bleeding. Take a sexual history to find out about contraception use, recent partners, any previous history of sexually transmitted infections, and any high risk sexual behaviour e.g. unprotected intercourse with multiple recent partners. Perform a systemic enquiry to identify any other symptoms that may help to localise an infective source for her pyrexia.
Examine the patient's abdomen to assess for tenderness. Perform a speculum vaginal examination and take "triple swabs" and perform a bimanual pelvic examination to assess for cervical excitation, adnexal masses/tenderness and

CLINICAL

uterine tenderness. Perform a general examination to look for other localising signs of infection e.g. a rash or chest signs.

As the patient is pyrexial her acute management should include the initial management of sepsis. Namely, she should have blood cultures taken, her urine output measured, intravenous fluids and antibiotics commenced, and serum lactate should be checked.

What investigations would aid your diagnosis

A pregnancy test is important to perform in women of reproductive age presenting with acute pain
Urine dip and microscopy and culture
FBC/U&Es/CRP
Blood cultures
Venous blood gas for lactate
"Triple swabs": a high vaginal swab for culture, an endocervical swab for culture, and a chlamydia swab
Consider a pelvic ultrasound: this is to look to for other causes of pelvic pain rather than detecting PID

What is the definition of PID?

Infection ascending from the endocervix to affect the pelvis resulting in endometritis, parametritis, salpingitis, oophoritis and/or pelvic peritonitis i.e. inflammation of the reproductive organs and lining of the pelvis. Tubo-ovarian abscesses can also occur with PID.

What would be the next steps in managing a patient with PID?

The patient should be advised that referral to a Genito-Urinary Medicine (GUM) clinic is recommended. Self referral is usually possible. Treatment for PID should be commenced if she is not already on empirical antibiotics. Contact tracing should be performed and sexual health screening to check for other sexually transmitted infections e.g. HIV should be offered. These services can be provided via the GUM clinic. The patient (and her partner) should not have unprotected sexual intercourse until treatment and follow up is completed.

What long term consequences of PID would you counsel patients about?

The long term complications of PID include an increased risk of ectopic pregnancy and subfertility. More chronic pelvic pain can also occur.

What organisms cause PID?

Neisseria gonorrhoea and Chlamydia trachomatis are both causes. Gardnerella vaginalis and anaerobic organisms may also be causative organisms. Mycoplasma genitalium is also associated with upper genital tract infection in women.

What antibiotics would you use to treat PID as an inpatient?

An evidence based regime would be giving IV ceftriaxone and IV doxycycline

CLINICAL

and continuing these until 24 hours after clinical improvement. Oral metronidazole should also be started. Once IV therapy is no longer needed oral doxycycline should be given and metronidazole continued and the doxycycline and metronidazole courses should be for a total of 2 weeks.

It is important to check local guidelines for variation based on availability of medicines and local antibiotic resistance patterns.

When would you suggest removal of an intra-uterine contraceptive device (IUCD) in a woman with PID?

The decision to remove an IUCD should consider the relative merits of helping to treat the PID versus the loss of contraception, both in the immediate and longer term. If an IUCD is to be removed then consideration to other forms of contraception, including any need for emergency contraception, should be given. It is reasonable to remove an IUCD if:

The woman requests it

There is no clinical improvement after 72 hours of treatment

The patient has pelvic pain, and there is a history of actinomyces-like organisms on cervical smear

SUMMARY

There are many causes of abdominal pain in women of reproductive age and this can make diagnosing PID difficult. Clinical symptoms and signs may not be specific to PID. In addition, negative swabs do not exclude PID. It is therefore important to have a low threshold for considering the diagnosis of PID and commencing PID treatment in sexually active women. PID can have significant long term complications and the chances of these occurring is reduced if treatment is started promptly.

TOP TIPS

 Remember that a sexual history, and pelvic examination, can be sensitive topics for patients and consider the privacy of where you are seeing the patient. A single room rather than a curtained bay is preferable.

References:
British Association for Sexual Health and HIV- UK National Guideline for the Management of Pelvic Inflammatory Disease 2011

3.10 Hypertension (1)

Scenario

A 40-year-old woman presents to the day assessment unit at 36/40 complaining of feeling generally unwell with reflux and leg swelling. This is her first pregnancy. You note that she is hypertensive at 155/98. You have been asked to review her.

What is your differential diagnosis?

Pre-eclampsia
Pregnancy induced hypertension
Essential hypertension
HELLP syndrome
DVT
Oedema of pregnancy
Reflux of pregnancy
Gastritis/hiatus hernia/IBS
In this scenario the most important feature of note is that the patient is hypertensive at 155/98. This is a significantly raised blood pressure. This high blood pressure in combination with her symptoms suggests the likely diagnosis being pre-eclampsia and the clinician should be very aware of this diagnosis. A review of the notes will inform you if she has had any previous high blood pressure readings or a background of essential hypertension before.

How would you acutely manage this patient?

The first thing to do is an ABCD assessment.
Once the patient is identified as stable a detailed history and examination should be performed.

The history should identify any risk factors for pre-eclampsia or other symptoms/signs of pre-eclampsia.

Examination should feature palpation of the abdomen to assess symphysis fundal height and auscultating the fetal heart rate. Assessment of reflexes and examination for clonus is important. Some clinicians suggest examining for papilloedema and auscultating the chest to exclude pulmonary oedema.

Initial management should include blood tests, urinalysis (protein:creatinine ratio) and CTG in the antenatal setting after 28/40. If the patient is thought to have pre-eclampsia they need very close observation and consideration for delivery made in combination with the obstetric team. This depends on the clinical situation and the gestation and well being of the fetus.

What investigation would aid your diagnosis

Bloods: FBC, U&Es, LFTs, uric acid- clotting studies should also be performed

CLINICAL

if platelets are less than 100
Ultrasound scan: assessment of fetal size, umbilical artery dopplers and liquor volume – risk of reduced end diastolic flow, IUGR (in 30% of pre-eclamptic cases) and stillbirth
Leg venous dopplers: DVT
AXR/endoscopy: non-pregnancy related abdominal pain

Define the epidemiology of pre-eclampsia

Pre-eclampsia affects approximately 2-8% pregnancies and is severe in 0.5% of cases.

What is the classification of raised blood pressure in pregnancy?

Severe: 160/110
Moderate: 150/100
Mild: 140/90
Pregnancy induced hypertension: hypertension in the absence of proteinuria
Pre-eclampsia: hypertension in the presence of proteinuria (PCR>30)
HELLP: haemolysis, elevated liver enzymes and low platelets

Outline the symptoms of pre-eclampsia

- Headache
- Altered vision
- Epigastric pain
- Vomiting
- Clonus
- Papilloedema
- Liver tenderness
- Reflex
- Facial oedema

What are the risk factors of pre-eclampsia and what is the mainstay of risk reduction?

- Primip
- 40 years old or over
- Pregnancies 10 or more years apart
- Raised BMI
- Family history of pre-eclampsia
- Multiple gestation
- Essential hypertension
- Previous pre-eclampsia
- Previous medical history of kidney disorder, diabetes, autoimmune condition (e.g. lupus)
- Aspirin 75mg once daily

Outline the antenatal management of pregnancy induced hypertension and pre-eclampsia

- **Pregnancy induced hypertension**
  - Aim for delivery at 37 weeks via induction or caesarean
  - Monitor if mild, treat as outpatient if moderate, treat as inpatient if severe
  - Repeat blood pressure monitoring once a week if mild, twice a week if moderate and four times daily if severe with urinalysis each visit/daily, both twice weekly if managing severe cases in community
  - Bloods once if moderate and no new proteinuria, weekly if severe/mild before 32 weeks/high risk

- **Pre-eclampsia**
  - Aim for delivery beyond 34 weeks if severe, if mild or moderate aim for 37 weeks
  - Admit all cases, treat if moderate or severe with four times daily blood pressure monitoring
  - No need to repeat urinalysis
  - Twice weekly monitoring of all cases in community

- **Consultant led care**
- **Medication**: labetalol *(methyldopa if asthmatic)*, nifedipine MR second line or combination, IV labetalol/hydralazine if refractory
  - Magnesium sulphate if eclampsia concerns

SUMMARY

Pre-eclampsia occurs beyond 20 weeks of pregnancy (usually essential hypertension prior to this), and is characterised by hypertension and proteinuria. It has been heavily featured in recent MBRRACE reports and should be considered a serious complication of pregnancy and managed as such. Hypertension and fits in pregnancy should be managed as pre-eclampsia/eclampsia until proven otherwise.

TOP TIPS

 Speed of administration of medication is paramount in this station, particularly in severe cases. Do not wait on additional results such as urine dip/bloods before initiating your management plan. It is likely that the interviewers will be looking for your regard of the seriousness of the situation and potentially calling for help if eclampsia appears imminent as opposed to asking the patient about her pre-eclampsia risk factors, manage it as such.

3.11 Sepsis

Scenario

A 34-year-old woman has returned to the ward after being discharged home 1 day ago following an uncomplicated spontaneous vaginal delivery at term. She complains of feeling generally unwell with hot flushes and some mild abdominal pain. She is febrile with a tachycardia. You have been asked to review her.

What is your differential diagnosis?

Endometritis
Mastitis
Skin and soft tissue infection
Urinary tract infection
Pneumonia
Gastroenteritis
Pharyngitis
Infection related to regional anaesthesia
The most common site of sepsis in the puerperium is the genital tract, and in particular the uterus, resulting in endometritis.

How would you acutely manage this patient?

This patient should be stabilised with an ABCDE approach, including assessment of the airway, respiratory and circulatory system as well as conscious level. Once the patient is identified as stable a detailed history and examination should be performed.

Airway: Examine for signs of airway obstruction such as stridor or noisy breathing. Assess patients ability to talk in full sentences.

Breathing: Respiratory rate, oxygen saturations. Auscultate lung fields. Supply patient with high flow oxygen (15L) via a non-rebreathe mask. High flow oxygen should be administered to all acutely ill patients.

Circulation: Assess blood pressure, capillary refill time, heart rate and rhythm. We have been informed that this patient is tachycardic so it is appropriate to insert two large bore cannulas and commence fluid challenges titrated to the patients response. Whilst inserting the cannula draw off bloods including blood cultures, FBC, U+Es, LFTs CRP and venous lactate. Examine for circulatory features of septic shock including warm peripheries and a bounding pulse. Hourly fluid balance including urine output should be monitored.

Disability: Examine conscious level using AVPU or GCS scoring system.

Exposure: Examine for other signs that might identify the source of this patients fever and tachycardia. Commence analgesia to ensure the patient is comfortable. Look for signs of organ dysfunction.

What investigations would aid your diagnosis?

Blood cultures: these should be taken immediately and prior to antibiotic administration.
Serum lactate: should be measured within 6 hours of the suspicion of severe sepsis. Lactate ≥ 4 mmol/l is indicative of tissue hypoperfusion.
Imaging: this might include CXR, or pelvic USS/CT scan if you are considering an abdominal collection or abscess.
Baseline bloods: FBC U+E CRP.
Vaginal swab: if patient can tolerate a high vaginal swab this is preferable to a low vaginal swab.
Any woman with a history of a sore throat should have a throat swab taken.
Midstream urine
Expressed breast milk swab
Stool for culture if diarrhoea present
Nose swab for MRSA screening.
Check for placental swab results.

What is the definition of sepsis in the puerperium?

Sepsis developing after birth until 6 weeks postnatally.

Which antibiotics should be used?

High dose intravenous broad spectrum antibiotics should be started within one hour and without waiting for results if sepsis is suspected. Once an infection becomes systemic the woman's condition can deteriorate rapidly. Abdominal pain, fever and tachycardia are indications for intravenous antibiotics.
The RCOG suggests a combination of Tazocin plus clindamycin provides one of the broadest ranges of treatment for severe sepsis.
The choice of antibiotics should be guided by hospital policy and microbiologist input.

What are some common organisms causing infection in the puerperium?

Group A streptococcus (also known as streptococcus pyogenes)
Escherichia Coli
Staphylococcus aureus
Methicillin resistant staphylococcus aureus
Group A streptococcus is increasingly causing invasive infections worldwide and was directly responsible for causing 13 of the 29 deaths from infection in the UK between 2006-2008 (CMACE 2011).

What are some risk factors for sepsis in the puerperium?

Obesity
Impaired glucose tolerance / diabetes

CLINICAL

Anaemia
Vaginal trauma, tears and episiotomies
Prolonged spontaneous ruptured membranes
Retained products of conception /incomplete placenta
Invasive procedures, if a caesarean section was performed then this is a risk factor, other invasive procedures include epidural /amniocentesis /cervical cerclage
Group A streptococcus infection in close contact / family members

What are some examination signs of sepsis?

Pyrexia >38
Sustained tachycardia
Breathlessness with raised RR
Uterine tenderness, with possible raised symphysis fundal height if retained products suspected
Cellulitis, check breasts and vaginal tears/episiotomies for this
Vaginal discharge (try to perform speculum if tolerated)

How should this woman be monitored?

Monitoring should be performed in a multi-disciplinary team under the leadership of a single consultant. A senior obstetrician should always be involved in consultation with an intensivist and microbiologist.
Regular observations of all vital signs should be recorded on a modified early obstetric warning score (MEOWS) chart.
Handover should be robust.
Regular contact with family members is required.

What are the indications for admission to the intensive care unit?

Answer this questions with a structure, the best way to do this is to go through body systems and discuss each one.

Cardiovascular: Hypotension or raised serum lactate persisting despite fluid resuscitation suggesting the need for inotrope support.
Respiratory: Pulmonary oedema Mechanical ventilation Airway protection.
Renal: Renal dialysis.
Neurological: Significantly decreased conscious level.
Miscellaneous: Multi-organ failure, uncorrected acidosis, hypothermia.

What infectious disease history should be noted?

A history of recent sore throat or prolonged contact with family members with known streptococcal infection have been implicated in cases of known streptococcus.
Intravenous drug use – carries a high risk of staphylococcus and streptococcal sepsis.
Ingestions of unpasteurised milk raises the possibility of infection with salmonella, campylobacter or listeria.

CLINICAL

What is the role of intravenous immunoglobulin IVIG?

IVIG has an immunomodulatory effect. It is effective in exotoxic shock (toxic shock attributable to streptococci and staphylococci) but there is little evidence of benefit in gram negative sepsis.

SUMMARY

The most common sight of sepsis in the puerperium is the genital tract, resulting in endometritis. Group A Streptococcus (GAS) is one causative agent associated with a high mortality rate, it should be considered in all cases of sepsis. Screen for risk factors for GAS including previous sore throat and take a high vaginal and throat swab. Symptoms of sepsis may be less distinctive in a postnatal patient and so a high index of suspicion is indicated. There are many other causes of sepsis in the post-natal period and you should demonstrate that you are aware of these by asking about them in your history and examination (mastitis, urinary tract infection, pneumonia, skin and soft-tissue infection, gastroenteritis, pharyngitis, infection related to regional anaesthesia). Blood cultures should be taken first and broad spectrum antibiotics started within one hour if sepsis is suspected.

TOP TIPS

➕ Do not forget to ask the patient if they have any allergies. It is very likely that in this station you will be asked what antibiotics to prescribe for sepsis. You must consider the patients allergies before responding to this.

➕ When examining for endometritis do not forget to perform a vaginal and abdominal examination. On abdominal examination you are looking for a tender and bulky uterine fundus which might suggest retained products with superimposed infection. A speculum vaginal examination is preferable if this is tolerated by the patient. You should try to identify the cervix for offensive discharge. A high vaginal swab should be taken. At the same time any tears/episotomy wounds should be examined.

➕ Make sure you listen carefully to the patient. For example do not ask about healing of the caesarean scar if they had a spontaneous vaginal delivery.

CLINICAL

References
Centre for Maternal and Child Enquiries (CMACE). Saving Mothers' Lives: reviewing maternal deaths to make motherhood safer: 2006–08.
The Eighth Report on Confidential Enquiries into Maternal Deaths in the United Kingdom. BJOG 2011;118 Suppl 1:1–203.

3.12 Post-Partum Haemorrhage (PPH) (1)

> ### Scenario
> You are asked to urgently review a 26-year-old lady in the labour room by the midwife who reports rapid blood loss immediately following a spontaneous vaginal delivery.

What is your differential diagnosis?

Tone: uterine atony, distended bladder.
Trauma: lacerations of the uterus, cervix, or vagina.
Tissue: retained placenta or clots.
Thrombin: pre-existing or acquired coagulopathy.

The most common reason for primary PPH is uterine atony, followed by retained placenta or clots.

How would you acutely manage this patient?

Management of PPH has 4 broad components: communication with all relevant professionals; resuscitation; monitoring and investigation and measures to arrest the bleeding. These must be initiated and progressed simultaneously for optimal patient care.

Resuscitation
Airway and Breathing: assess airway and breathing A high concentration of oxygen (10–15 litres/minute) via a facemask should be administered, regardless of maternal oxygen concentration. If the airway is compromised, anaesthetic assistance should be sought urgently.

Circulation: Establish two large bore cannulae; 20 ml blood sample should be taken and sent. Transfuse blood as soon as possible. Until blood is available, infuse up to 3.5 litres of warmed crystalloid Hartmann's solution (2 litres) and/or colloid (1-2 litres) as rapidly as required.

Disability: Position flat. Monitor conscious level using AVPU or GCS scoring system

Exposure: Examine to assess tone of uterus and exclude other sources of bleeding. Keep the woman warm using appropriate available measures.

Monitoring
Blood: crossmatch (4 units minimum), full blood count, coagulation screen including fibrinogen, renal and liver function for baseline.
Monitor temperature every 15 minutes.
Continuous HR, BP and %O2 sats monitoring.
Catheterise to monitor urine output.

Consider arterial line monitoring.
Consider transfer to ITU once the bleeding is controlled or monitoring at HDU on delivery suite.
Recording of parameters on a flow chart such as the modified obstetric early warning system charts.
Documentation of fluid balance, blood, blood products and procedures.

Arresting the bleeding
The most common cause of primary post-partum haemorrhage is uterine atony. Examine to exclude the following: Retained products (placenta, membranes, clots), vaginal/cervical lacerations or haematoma, ruptured uterus, broad ligament haematoma, uterine inversion, extragenital bleeding (e.g subcapsular liver rupture).
When uterine atony is perceived to be a cause of the bleeding, the following mechanical and pharmacological measures should be instituted, in turn, until the bleeding stops:
Bimanual uterine compression (rubbing up the fundus) to stimulate contractions.
Ensure bladder is empty (Foley catheter, leave in place).
Syntocinon 5 units by slow intravenous injection (may have repeat dose).
Ergometrine 0.5 mg by slow intravenous or intramuscular injection (contraindicated in women with hypertension).
Syntocinon infusion (40 units in 500 ml Hartmann's solution at 125 ml/hour) unless fluid restriction is necessary.
Carboprost 0.25 mg by intramuscular injection repeated at intervals of not less than 15 minutes to a maximum of 8 doses (contraindicated in women with asthma).
Direct intramyometrial injection of carboprost 0.5 mg (contraindicated in women with asthma), with responsibility of the administering clinician as it is not recommended for intramyometrial use.
Misoprostol 1000 micrograms rectally.

What investigations could aid your diagnosis?

Crossmatch: 4 units minimum
Bloods: FBC to assess Hb in comparison to antenatal, platelet count, urea and electrolytes, liver function tests
Coagulation screen including fibrinogen: to assess need for FFP and cryoprecipitate

If pharmacological management of PPH fails, what surgical options are available?

- Intrauterine balloon tamponade
- Haemostatic brace suturing *(such as using procedures described by B-Lynch or modified compression sutures)*, bilateral ligation of uterine arteries
- Bilateral ligation of internal iliac *(hypogastric)* arteries
- Selective arterial embolization
- Hysterectomy

Name 5 key risk factors for PPH which are may be known about antenatally

Placenta accreta/percreta
Placental abruption
Placenta praevia
Multiple pregnancy
Pre-eclampsia
Previous PPH
Asian ethnicity
Obesity: BMI>35
Anaemia: Hb < 9

Name 5 key risk factors for PPH which may present themselves during labour

EMCS
Elective CS
IOL
Retained placenta
Mediolateral episiotomy
Operative vaginal delivery
Prolonged labour >12 hours
Big baby > 4kg
Pyrexia in labour
Age > 40 years

Obstetrically, what is the main method by which PPH is prevented?

Active management of the 3rd stage of labour.
Active management of the third stage of labour lowers maternal blood loss and reduces the risk of PPH. Prophylactic oxytocics are offered to all women as they reduce the risk of PPH by about 60%. For women without risk factors for PPH delivering vaginally, oxytocin (5 iu or 10 iu by intramuscular injection) is first line.

What are the broad definitions for minor vs. major PPH?

Minor PPH: Blood loss 500-1000mls, no clinical signs of shock
Major PPH: Blood loss > 1000mls and continuing to bleed or signs of clinical shock.

How should secondary PPH be managed?

Secondary PPH is often associated with endometritis. Prompt administration of antibiotics and 'sepsis 6' are paramount to management. Surgical measures should be undertaken if there is excessive or continuing bleeding. A senior obstetrician should be involved in decisions and performance of any evacuation of retained products of conception as uterus is very friable postpartum.

What are the main complications of continued, severe PPH?

Hypovolaemic shock

Disseminated intravascular coagulation
Renal and liver failure
ARDS
Death

What is DIC and how is it diagnosed?

Disseminated intravascular coagulation (DIC) is a consumptive coagulopathy. Widespread activation of the clotting cascade that results in the formation of blood clots in the small blood vessels. This leads to compromise of tissue blood flow and can rapidly progress to multiple organ failure. As the coagulation process consumes clotting factors and platelets, severe bleeding can occur from various sites. Blood markers include a prolonged PT, aPTT and rapidly decreasing platelet count. D-dimer is raised.

SUMMARY

Primary post-partum haemorrhage is primarily due to one of the 4T's: tone, tissue,trauma, thrombin. PPH is frequently prevented by active management of the 3rd stage of labour with oxytocin. It can be defined as minor – blood loss 500-1000mls with no signs of hypovolemic shock or major >1000mls with continuing bleeding and/or signs of shock. Risk factors for PPH may be present antenatally or develop during labour for example undergoing a mediolateral episiotomy or retained placenta. Patients with PPH should be managed with a ABCDE approach, the RCOG recommends simultaneous communication, resuscitation, investigation and monitoring and actions to arrest the bleeding as effective management. Complications of PPH include hypovolaemic shock, DIC, multiorgan failure and death. Early involvement of senior members of staff and anaesthetic support is crucial.

CLINICAL

TOP TIPS

+ Emphasis is required on effective resuscitation using a structured ABCDE description.

+ Good knowledge is required of the causes of PPH and how these may be managed more specifically.

+ Don't forget to research in more detail surgical techniques for management of PPH in order to describe why they are often effective.

3.13 Fetal Distress (1)

Scenario

You are the SHO on labour ward when the emergency alarm sounds; you are directed to room 3. There is a 28-year-old primip, with an uncomplicated obstetric history, who on last assessment 2 hours ago was 6cm dilated. As you head towards the room, the midwife opens the door and says the baseline rate is 60bpm.

What is your differential diagnosis?

Fetal bradycardia

It is important to clearly state the nature of the emergency to anyone arriving in an emergency situation. This reduces confusion and improves team-working to deal with it. Fetal bradycardia is a common emergency to take place on labour ward and though it often resolves spontaneously, needs to be dealt with appropriately and promptly.

How would you acutely manage this patient?

A quick ABCDE assessment of the mother should be done.

Airway: introducing yourself and talking will confirm her airway.

Breathing: an oxygen saturation probe, often used to record her pulse, will give you a quick assessment of saturations for breathing.

Circulation: note her pulse; it must be differentiated from the fetal heart, and may be causing fetal abnormalities (e.g. maternal tachycardia is often mirrored with fetal tachycardia). IV access should be inserted, full blood count and group and save sent urgently, and recent blood pressure reading checked.

Disability: assess using AVPU

Exposure: check the temperature, and any other concerns.

If there are any problems with any stages, then a full detailed ABCDE assessment needs to be performed.

Whilst doing this brief assessment it is important to also assess the fetal situation simultaneously. The CTG should be reviewed, including previous periods of recording to note how it has changed over time. If it is a true fetal bradycardia then prompt action is needed.
Initially, conservative measures should be used: changing position – first into left lateral, and then right lateral, IV fluids should be commenced and run straight through, contractions should be reviewed, and any oxytocin should be stopped

CLINICAL

and tocolysis considered. Seniors should be alerted: obstetric registrar or consultant, labour ward co-ordinator, anaesthetist and theatre teams. A vaginal examination should be performed to assess progress, ensure there is no cord prolapse, and plan for delivery.

The 'rule of 3' can be used to ensure delivery is expedited in a timely manner if the baseline rate does not improve: 3 minutes: call for help, 6 minutes: transfer to theatre clearly calling it as a category 1 LSCS, 9 minutes: prepare for assisted delivery, 12 minutes: aim to deliver baby.

What investigations would aid your diagnosis

The bradycardia would be diagnosed on CTG. All other investigations are involved with managing the bradycardia rather than diagnosing it.

What is the definition of fetal bradycardia?

A single prolonged deceleration with baseline below 100 bpm, persisting for 3 minutes or more.

What are possible causes of fetal bradycardia?

Placental abruption: a large abruption can interrupt perfusion of the fetus and cause an acute bradycardia.

Severe PET: this may be preceded by other signs of fetal distress, often due to placental insufficiency. PET may also cause an abruption, then causing bradycardia.

Cord prolapse: this is a rare but important cause of bradycardia, and should be assessed on vaginal examination. If there is cord present, efforts should be made to lift the baby up off the cord to release compression whilst plan for delivery is made.

Uterine rupture: this is rare but an increasing factor as the LSCS rate rises. Constant, severe pain across the scar should not be ignored, and can lead to acute fetal compromise.

Cord compression: this is a common cause of decelerations in labour, particularly in the second stage but they are often not pathological. As labour progresses, they may become more pronounced and if not managed appropriately lead to bradycardia. Equally, if the cord is wrapped around the baby, descent can cause increasing compression which will not recover and cause bradycardia.

Sepsis: of the mother or the fetus can lead to fetal distress. There is likely to be a step-wise deterioration, but if untreated will lead to bradycardia.

Poor reserve for labour: antenatal risk factors may make a fetus more likely to deteriorate in labour. There is normally evidence of progressive deterioration, but if this is not correctly identified and managed it may finally result in bradycardia.

How is classification of urgency of Caesarean section defined?

The basic classification of LSCS is into emergency vs elective. Commonly units also use a category classification:

- **Category 1**: Immediate threat to life of mother of fetus. For audit targets this is usually <30 minutes but many units aim for delivery within 15 mins.

CLINICAL

- **Category 2**: No immediate threat to life of mother or fetus, but presence of maternal or fetal compromise.
- **Category 3**: Requires early delivery, may be some evidence of maternal or fetal compromise.
- **Category 4** *(Elective)*: At a time to suit mother and maternity services, no fetal or maternal compromise.
- Most units have timings for delivery for each category, but these vary.

SUMMARY

Fetal bradycardia is a true obstetric emergency and needs to be dealt with promptly and appropriately. Wasting time can cause acute hypoxia of the fetus leading to acidosis and potentially permanent damage and finally death. It can be very distressing for the mother and her partner, and it is important to explain what is happening and keep them informed. Appropriate consent (ideally written) should be gained before procedures are performed, and debriefing is an important part of the management. Appropriate training for fetal bradycardia should be done regularly by the whole multidisciplinary team (e.g. PROMPT) to improve management.

TOP TIPS

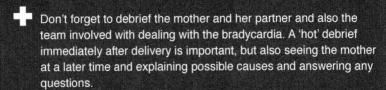 Don't forget to debrief the mother and her partner and also the team involved with dealing with the bradycardia. A 'hot' debrief immediately after delivery is important, but also seeing the mother at a later time and explaining possible causes and answering any questions.

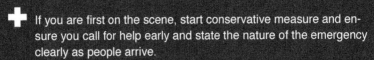 If you are first on the scene, start conservative measure and ensure you call for help early and state the nature of the emergency clearly as people arrive.

References:
Classification of Urgency of Caesarean Risk, Royal College of Obstetricians and Gynaecologists, Good Practice No. 11, April 2010

Interpretation of Cardiotocograph Traces, Intrapartum Care, NICE guideline CG190, Dec 2014

3.14 | Post-Menopausal Bleeding

Scenario

A 55-year-old-female has come to clinic after a 2-week wait referral from her GP with a 1-week history of heavy postmenopausal bleeding. You know her last menstrual period was aged 50; she has no previous history of menorrhagia and is not on any hormone replacement therapy. You have been asked to review her and suggest a management plan. As you walk over to her you think she looks quite pale and may be about to faint.

What is your differential diagnosis?

Endometrial cancer or hyperplasia
Atrophic vaginitis
Endometrial or endocervical polyp
Cervical or ovarian cancer
Iatrogenic (HRT withdrawal, anticoagulation)

The large majority (90%) of post-menopausal bleeding (PMB) is due to benign causes. However as 5-10% is due to endometrial cancer, PMB should be considered worrying until proven otherwise. Any vaginal bleeding after the menopause is abnormal. Factors within the history can help to distinguish high-risk cases. Any personal or family history of endometrial, breast or ovarian cancer will increase clinical suspicion of cancer. Obese women (BMI >25) are twice as likely to develop the disease; the likelihood of more serious disease increases with age, average age of presentation of endometrial cancer is 60. Drug use – such as HRT or Tamoxifen increases risk of benign or malignant endometrial tumours. Withdrawal from HRT and anticoagulant use can cause iatrogenic bleeding.

How would you acutely manage this patient?

This patient in this scenario looks quite unwell from the end of the bed so could have had significant blood loss. It is therefore important to approach her with an acute management plan

Airway: ensure remains patent, if the patient is likely to faint in clinic, move her to a bed, or if on the floor into the recovery position, suction may be required if the patient vomits.

Breathing: check observations such as respiratory rate and oxygen saturations, and examine the chest. If she becomes acutely unwell she may need oxygen so make sure a supply is available.

Circulation: extreme vaginal blood loss can cause anaemia, if the patient has not replaced fluids dehydration and even hypovolaemic shock could occur. Heart rate and rhythm, heart sounds, temperature, blood pressure and capil-

CLINICAL

lary refill time should be checked. If fluid replacement is needed two large bore cannulas should be inserted and fluid challenge given. Blood tests will probably be needed, FBC to assess level of anaemia, clotting screen, to look at bleeding risk and for any coagulopathies or bleeding conditions, U+Es to check for dehydration, as well as a group and save if the patient is heading for a blood transfusion.

Disability: the patient should not be left alone, close monitoring of consciousness using GCS/AVPU, a blood glucose level should be taken if indicated.

Exposure: confirm blood loss is vaginal in origin or other potential causes of collapse such as infection.

What investigations would aid your diagnosis?

When investigating post-menopausal bleeding investigations could be requested in the following order:

Bloods: FBC to assess anaemia. If the patient is stable, only need other tests such as clotting and endocrine tests if the history is suggestive
Transvaginal Ultra Sound (TVS): 1st line imaging. Endometrial thickness <5mm is associated with normal endometrial atrophy and reduces the likelihood of malignant disease to <2%. Most women with disease such as endometrial hyperplasia, polyps or submucous fibroids will have an increased thickness >5mm, which will require further investigation by Endometrial biopsy and/or Hysteroscopy.
Cervical smear: if not done recently, to look for cervical cancer. If cytology shows atypical glandular endometrial sampling should also be done.
Endometrial biopsy: if any increased endometrial thickness. Highly reliable with sensitivity >99%, it confirms histology and can identify tumour grade and subtype, however has a failure rate of 10% of getting a sufficient sample.
Outpatient hysteroscopy or dilatation and curettage: gold standard focal intrauterine pathology or significant endometrial disease suspected, with samples sent for histology
MRI/CT: imaging indicated for staging if endometrial/cervical cancer

How is post-menopausal bleeding defined?

Any vaginal bleeding that occurs 12 months or more after a woman's last menstrual cycle.
This is not to be confused with peri-menstrual bleeding – many women will have irregular cycles in the run up to the menopause, they may go several months amenorrhoeic and then have a normal cycle with a bleed. The menopause can only be confirmed once 12 months of amenorrhoea have passed without the use of hormonal contraception.

What is the management and prognosis for Stage 1 endometrial cancer?

Total abdominal hysterectomy and bilateral salping-oophorectomy – 90% of women present with early disease. Less commonly if disease present late ad-

junct radiotherapy may be needed
Prognosis is good for stage 1 with >70% 5 year survival

SUMMARY

Post-menopausal bleeding is a common complaint, and can require referral to secondary care. A full gynaecological and obstetric history should be taken to determine LMP and menarche to confirm post-menopausal then careful history to determine other relevant symptoms. Unless the patient is haemodynamically unstable or other symptoms are present, only an FBC is required, most patients will need to be referred from their GP for TVS under 2 week wait unless examination confirms the definitive source for the bleeding. Many women will be worried about cancer and it is difficult to reassure them until the results of all required further investigations are back, however the majority of causes and benign and easily treated.

TOP TIPS

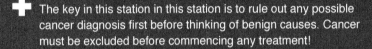 The key in this station in this station is to rule out any possible cancer diagnosis first before thinking of benign causes. Cancer must be excluded before commencing any treatment!

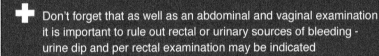 Don't forget that as well as an abdominal and vaginal examination it is important to rule out rectal or urinary sources of bleeding - urine dip and per rectal examination may be indicated

CLINICAL

References:
Clark, T. Justin, and Janesh Kumar Gupta. Handbook Of Outpatient Hysteroscopy: A Complete Guide to Diagnosis and Therapy. London: Hodder Arnold, 2005

3.15   Abdo Pain and Bleeding in Labour

Scenario

You are asked to review a lady on the labour ward. She has had one previous caesarean section and is in spontaneous labour. The midwife has asked you to see her as the patient is reporting new abdominal pain though her contractions seem to have abruptly stopped, and there has been some vaginal blood loss.

What is your differential diagnosis?

Uterine rupture
Placental abruption
Vasa praevia
Placenta praevia minor
Uterine hyperstimulation

How would you acutely manage this patient?

The patient should be managed with an ABCDE approach to determine how clinically stable she is.

Airway and Breathing: Establish that the airway is maintained and there are no concerns with breathing.

Circulation: Site at least one large cannula (16G or larger) and start intravenous fluids if the patient is tachycardic and hypotensive.

Disability: Assess the patient's responsiveness using AVPU or the GCS and then once the patient is stable take a history.

Exposure: Determine the duration, location and character of the patient's pain, paying particular attention to if the pain is constant. Determine the volume of vaginal bleeding and when it started.

Find out the background of the patient's labour so far including her progress in labour (dilatation at last vaginal examination) and whether any intervention e.g. oxytocin has been used, or if the patient is having an induction of labour. Review the patient's previous deliveries to find out the indication for her previous caesarean and any other deliveries she has had. In practice this can be done by reviewing her maternity notes rather than using direct questioning.

Examine the patient's abdomen to assess for contractions, the lie and presentation of the fetus, and engagement of the presenting part. Assess for areas of tenderness especially suprapubically over the previous caesarean scar. Also assess for any easily palpable fetal parts. After confirming that the placenta is not low lying, perform a vaginal examination to determine the dilatation of the cervix and the station and position of the presenting part. Patients in VBAC labour are usually monitored routinely with a cardiotocograph (CTG). Start CTG monitoring if this is not the case and review the CTG to assess the fetal heart rate for decelerations or bradycardia, and the contraction frequency.

After assessing the patient if the clinical impression is uterine rupture then immediate escalation to a senior would be appropriate, and consider if the patient needs transfer to the operating theatre for further management. Inform the multi-disciplinary team i.e. labour ward co-ordinator/anaesthetist/paediatrician of the plan.

What investigations would aid your diagnosis

Take blood for FBC and group and save/crossmatch when siting a cannula. If there are concerns with the amount of vaginal bleeding then a crossmatch is preferable, and U&Es and a coagulation screen would also be appropriate. The suspicion of uterine rupture in VBAC is ultimately a clinical one and investigations e.g. bloods should be aimed at preparing the patient for surgery. Continuous CTG monitoring.

What is the definition of uterine rupture?

A defect in the uterine wall including both the myometrial and serosal layers. Uterine dehiscence refers to a defect of the myometrium with an intact serosa.

How common is uterine rupture?

Uterine rupture in VBAC has an incidence of 0.5%. Uterine rupture in an unscarred uterus is much rarer, with an incidence of 1 in 5000 (0.02%).

What are the risk factors for uterine rupture?

Previous caesarean section
Augmentation/Induction of labour in VBAC
Previous uterine surgery
Previous uterine rupture
Inter-delivery interval less than 12 months
Macrosomia
Decreased lower uterine segment myometrial thickness on antenatal ultrasound

What are the contra-indications to VBAC?

Other pathology requiring delivery by caesarean section e.g. major placenta praevia
Previous classical caesarean section, or "inverted T" or "J" uterine incisions
Previous uterine rupture
More than one previous caesarean, although VBAC can be offered in this patient group after discussion with a senior obstetrician and counselling on risk of uterine rupture and morbidity, and provided the women delivers in a setting where facilities for immediate caesarean section, if necessary, are available.

CLINICAL

What success rates for VBAC would you counsel women about antenatally?

VBAC has a 72-75% success rate, but having a previous vaginal delivery, including previous successful VBAC, improve the chances to 85-90%.

How would you investigate for uterine rupture in a woman who has just delivered vaginally?

If uterine rupture is suspected in the late second stage of labour or with delivery, then an examination under anaesthetic can be undertaken in theatre to assess the integrity of the uterine scar. If a rupture is found, laparotomy to correct the defect would be needed.

SUMMARY

Uterine rupture is an obstetric emergency requiring prompt recognition of its symptoms and signs, and is a clinical diagnosis. Classically the presence of constant abdominal pain, vaginal bleeding and an abnormal fetal heart rate/pattern suggests uterine rupture. As caesarean section rates increase, a greater proportion of the obstetric patient population will be exposed to a risk of uterine rupture. In the future there may be a role for antenatal/intrapartum ultrasound assessment of the lower uterine segment to stratify risk of uterine scar rupture, but this needs evaluating. Women who have had a previous caesarean section or who have other risk factors for rupture need careful antenatal counselling so they know what to expect with VBAC labour.

TOP TIPS

➕ Remember to obtain the patient's past obstetric and gynaecological history as this will provide clues about her risk of uterine rupture.

➕ Remember that prompt escalation of the patient to a senior obstetrician and the labour ward multi-disciplinary team is important in obstetric emergencies, especially if theatre will be required.

➕ Obstetric emergencies are stressful for both the staff involved and patients and birth partners. Remember that part of the process of managing emergencies is to debrief with staff soon after the event to draw out any learning points. The woman and her birth partner should also have a debrief of what happened after the event.

References:
Royal College of Obstetricians and Gynaecologists Green Top Guideline Number 45 "Birth after Previous Caesarean Birth" (Published 01/10/2015)

3.16 | Acute Pelvic Pain (2)

Scenario

A 24-year-old woman presents to the emergency department with sudden onset vomiting and severe constant pain localised to the right iliac fossa (RIF) below McBurney's point. She no other symptoms. She has no relevant past medical, gynaecological or surgical history. She has a 28 day menstrual cycle, she is sexually active and has always used condoms for contraception. There is no vaginal bleeding. You have been asked to review her.

What is your differential diagnosis?

Ovarian torsion – cyst / idiopathic / neoplasm
Ovarian mass – cyst / neoplasm
Ruptured ovarian cyst
Ectopic pregnancy
Appendicitis
Mittelschmerz
Endometriosis
Pelvic inflammatory disease
Tubo-ovarian abscess
Renal colic
Adhesions

Ovarian torsion is the most likely diagnosis. This is twisting of the ovary on its pedicle preventing ovarian artery or venous flow, it is considered a gynaecological emergency in view of the potential to develop ovarian necrosis an it should always be considered in this setting. These patients should have early laparoscopic surgery to release the twisting and ensure viability of the ovary. In a woman of reproductive age, ovarian torsion is probably as a consequence of an ovarian cyst, particularly if the cyst is large >5cm. In premenarchal girls, ovarian torsion is usually idiopathic, and in post-menopausal woman it could be as a result of neoplasm.

How would you acutely manage this patient?

Assess the patient using the ABCDE approach.

Airway: Ask the patient a brief question to ascertain if they are able to complete full sentences, and therefore if the airway is patent. If not, look inside the mouth, listen for upper airway sounds, feel for breaths and manage findings appropriately, calling for help if necessary.

Breathing: Look for cyanosis, feel for chest expansion and listen to the lung fields. Measure respiratory rate and oxygen saturations. High flow oxygen (15L) via a non-rebreathe mask should be administered to all acutely ill patients.

CLINICAL

Circulation: Look for pallor, feel the pulse for rate and rhythm and listen to the heart. Measure blood pressure, capillary refill time and temperature. Insert a cannula and take bloods including FBC, U+Es, LFTs, CRP, venous lactate and group and saves. Examine for features of septic shock and complete the sepsis six with blood cultures, fluids, catheter and urine output measurements and antibiotics if appropriate.

Disability: Examine conscious level using AVPU or GCS scoring system. Measure blood glucose.

Exposure and everything else: Offer analgesia and antiemetics to ensure the patient is comfortable. Once the patient is identified as stable, a detailed history and full abdominal examination and bimanual examination should then be performed.

However, if suspicion for torsion is high there should be early discussion with the anaesthetist, gynaecology team and theatre teams about performing an emergency laparoscopy to prevent ovarian necrosis.

What investigations would aid your diagnosis?

Blood tests: FBC, U&Es, LFTs, CRP, blood cultures and lactate to examine for anaemia due to haemorrhage, markers of infection and sepsis, and to rule out urological and gastroenterological causes of the pain. Group and saves should also be taken to prepare for surgery. If malignancy is suspected, tumour markers can be sent.
Bedside tests: Beta-hCG to rule out pregnancy and urine dip to rule out urological causes of the pain.
Imaging: Transabdominal and transvaginal ultrasound are effective to confirm clinical suspicion of ovarian torsion. CT and MRI would show similar findings to ultrasound, but are more costly and CT has the added risk of radiation.

What are the risk factors for ovarian torsion?

The mechanism of torsion is mechanical, so risk factors are those that disrupt the normal lie of the ovary.

Ovarian mass: functional cyst, corpus luteum, benign or malignant tumour
Reproductive age: due to increased likelihood of developing a cyst
Pregnancy: due to the corpus luteum cyst and laxity of tissues supporting the ovaries
Ovarian induction: due to theca lutein cysts
Longer ligamental supports: especially in prepubertal girls
Congenital anatomical abnormalities: long fallopian tubes, absent mesosalpinx
Greater risk for the right ovary: 71% of torsions are right-sided due to a longer ligament and the sigmoid colon restricting movement of the left ovary (Pena et al., 2000)
High intensity exercise or suddenly increased intra-abdominal pressure: an inciting event for torsion

Prior ovarian torsion: approximately 11% recurrence risk (Tsafrir et al., 2012)

Which serum tumour markers would you request if a malignant ovarian tumour were suspected?

CA-125 is the main serum marker used for diagnosis and monitoring. CA 19-9, CA 15-3, CEA, AFP, Beta-hCG and other markers may be useful in certain sub-types to evaluate response to treatment.

What are the complications of ovarian torsion?
- Ovarian infarction
- Ovarian necrosis
- Local haemorrhage
- Infection
- Peritonitis
- Sepsis
- Ovarian loss
- Adhesions
- Chronic pain
- Infertility *(rare)*
- Pregnancy loss *(if pregnant)*
- Surgical complications, e.g. bleeding, proceeding to an open procedure, injury to surrounding structures
- Post-surgical complications, e.g. pain, nausea, wound infection, retention of necrotic tissue, thromboembolism

Describe the surgical management of ovarian torsion

A laparoscopic approach is routinely used unless there is suspicion of malignancy. Firstly ovarian viability is assessed by direct visualisation and examination. Initially blue/black coloured ovaries have been shown to regain function and should be preserved if possible. Signs of necrosis include loss of normal structure and a gelatinous consistency. Taking into account prior discussions with the patient, surgery can then proceed to the appropriate option; i) detorsion and ovarian conservation +/- cystectomy, ii) salpingo-oophorectomy – for postmenopausal women, a necrotic ovary or suspicion of malignancy. Further options include oophoropexy to prevent recurrence of torsion. Oophoropexy involves shortening the utero-ovarian ligament or a suture to fix the ovary to the utero-sacral ligament or another structure.

Which ligament(s) does the ovary typically rotate around in ovarian torsion?

The ovary typically twists around both the infundibulopelvic ligament and the utero-ovarian ligament.

SUMMARY

Ovarian torsion is one of the most common gynaecological emergencies. It is commonly misdiagnosed so should always be included as a differential if appropriate. A 2007 study has shown that correct pre-operative diagnosis was made in only 38% of a sample of 115 patients (Hiller et al., 2007). Torsion usually involves the ovary and fallopian tube, and results in compression of vessels and blockage of venous and lymphatic outflow, oedema and infarction. The primary risk factor for torsion is an ovarian mass that may be shown on ultrasound. Torsion has been recorded in polycystic ovarian syndrome, but often the mass of the ovary is so large that it becomes fixed in the pelvis and therefore less likely to rotate. Fixing of a mass due to adhesions (malignant, endometriosis, abscess, past surgery) makes the ovary less likely to rotate, although adhesions can also provide a new site around which the ovary can twist. An ovarian mass in a postmenopausal woman should raise the suspicion of malignancy. Diagnosis of torsion can only be confirmed at the time of surgery. Timely management with surgery prevents ovarian loss and other complications.

TOP TIPS

 Ovarian torsion often has a variable, non-specific presentation, and can happen at any stage of a woman's life – postmenopausal, in the reproductive ages, pregnancy, premenarchal and even in utero *(Sakala et al., 1991)*. For infants ask about feeding intolerance, vomiting, abdominal distension, and irritability. Do not be put off if pain radiates to the back, loin, groin or thigh, and if there is no palpable mass - ovarian torsion is still a possibility.

 Ask relevant questions in the history, do an abdominal examination, Beta-hCG and urine dip to rule out differentials. Support clinical suspicion of torsion with a bimanual examination, and the patient should be worked up for surgery with blood tests including group and saves. Ultrasound is the imaging modality of choice and is often as reliable as CT and MRI in diagnosing torsion.

References:
Hiller N., Appelbaum L., Simanovsky N., Lev-Sagi A., Aharoni D., Sella T.: CT features of adnexal torsion. AJR Am J Roentgenol. 2007;189(1):124.
Pena J.E., Ufberg D., Cooney N., and Denis A.L.: Usefulness of Doppler sonography in the diagnosis of ovarian torsion. Fertil. Steril. 2000;73:p1047-1050.
Sakala E.P., Leon Z.A., Rouse G.A.: Management of antenatally diagnosed fetal ovarian cysts. Obstet. Gynecol. Surv. 1991 Jul;46(7):407-14.

3.17 | Rupture of Membranes

Scenario

You are asked to review a primigravid woman who is 38 weeks pregnant and has presented to the Maternity Unit with new onset runny clear vaginal loss.

What is your differential diagnosis?

Spontaneous rupture of membranes (SROM)
"Show" (loss of cervical mucus plug)
Pelvic infection e.g. thrush
Urinary incontinence

How would you acutely manage this patient?

Begin with an ABCD approach. Once the patient's airway, breathing, circulation and consciousness have been assessed (e.g. the presence of a set of normal observations in a patient who looks well) take a history.

Determine the character of the vaginal loss to help to work out if it is likely to be liquor. Ask about the colour and viscosity of her vaginal loss. This will also help to determine if there is meconium staining of the liquor. Determine the time when the loss started. Ask about abdominal pains, as spontaneous labour may begin after SROM. Also ask about any reduced fetal movements and feverishness as these may alter the need for intervention. Determine if she has any urinary symptoms that may suggest infection, which may lead to urinary incontinence.

Perform an abdominal examination to assess the fetal lie and presentation, and engagement of the presenting part. Auscultate the fetal heart with a handheld doppler device or Pinard stethoscope. Usually in clinical practice this will have been performed by a midwife on admission.
If it is certain SROM has occurred based on the history and the woman's ongoing vaginal loss (which can be observed on a sanitary/maternity pad) do not perform a speculum examination. However, if there is any uncertainty a sterile speculum examination to look for pooling of liquor in the vagina should be offered to the patient. Unless there are contractions, a digital vaginal examination is not necessary.
If SROM is confirmed, review the woman's history to find out if she has known colonisation with group B streptococcus (GBS). This is usually detected on a vaginal or rectal swab or urine culture antenatally.

What investigation would aid your diagnosis

Sterile speculum examination is not always mandatory but can be useful if it is not obvious if SROM has occurred or not.
There are a number of tests that are commercially available that are designed

to help to diagnose SROM. The nitrazine test involves assessing the pH of the vaginal loss. Other tests involve taking a vaginal swab to look for certain compounds found in liquor. The use of such tests is not routine in diagnosing SROM at term.

Blood tests for maternal FBC/CRP are not routinely required, though if a speculum examination is performed it is common practice to take a high vaginal swab for culture at the same time.

How would you counsel women with prelabour SROM at term?

Once SROM is confirmed the risk of serious neonatal infection rises to 1%, from a background risk of 0.5% with intact membranes. However, approximately 60% of women with prelabour SROM at term will go into spontaneous labour within 24 hours of SROM. For those women that do not spontaneously labour, arranging induction of labour for 24 hours after SROM occurred is reasonable. This approach allows time for spontaneous labour to occur whilst also managing the increased infection risk. The patient does not need to remain in hospital whilst awaiting labour if she is clinically well.

How would you manage a patient who declined induction of labour?

Patients who choose not to have an induction of labour after 24 hours of SROM should be advised to monitor their temperature every 4 hours in the daytime and to monitor for any change to the colour or smell of their liquor. If the patient becomes pyrexial or their vaginal loss becomes offensive they should present to hospital. Patients should also be advised to report any reduced fetal movements immediately, and fetal movements and heart rate should be assessed every 24 hours. Sexual intercourse may be associated with an increased risk of infection and so the patient may wish to abstain whilst waiting for labour to start. Having a bath or shower does not increase the risk of infection and these can be continued.

What factors would make you consider immediate induction of labour with SROM at term?

Reduced fetal movements
Presence of meconium
GBS colonisation
Clinical concern about infection e.g. offensive vaginal loss, pyrexia
Other obstetric factors influencing timing of delivery e.g. hypertension/pre-eclampsia

How would you manage a woman with SROM and known GBS colonisation?

In this scenario it is reasonable to offer immediate induction of labour rather than waiting 24 hours, due to the risk of neonatal infection with GBS. The aim is to reduce the period of time during which the fetus is potentially exposed to GBS in the urogenital tract. Women with GBS bacteriuria in the pregnancy or a previous GBS affected baby should also be given intravenous antibiotic prophy-

CLINICAL

laxis (IAP) once SROM is confirmed until delivery. Women with GBS detected on a vaginal or rectal swab in the pregnancy should be offered IAP, though local protocols for IAP in this patient group are variable.

What management steps would you undertake if the patient was preterm?

If preterm prelabour rupture of membranes (PPROM) is diagnosed the patient should be admitted to hospital for observation, and commenced on oral erythromycin. If she is under 34 weeks pregnant a course of antenatal steroids would be appropriate. Induction of labour between 34 and 37 weeks gestation would be appropriate though the exact timing within this period is contentious and relates to the need to balance the risks of preterm birth with the risk of infection.

SUMMARY

SROM at term is diagnosed based on the history and assessment of vaginal loss. This does not always mean a speculum examination is necessary. Management centres around timely intervention to manage the risk of infection with ruptured membranes balanced against the likelihood of the woman going into spontaneous labour. Various factors influence the exact timing of induction of labour but if there are no other concerns then awaiting the onset of spontaneous labour for 24 hours then proceeding to induction of labour is appropriate.

CLINICAL

TOP TIPS

➕ Remember to take a patient centred approach when discussing options and risks with patients, particularly if patients wish to deviate from prescribed pathways of care.

➕ Consider carefully whether any vaginal examinations are necessary when reviewing pregnant/labouring women. A vaginal examination should provide information that will change management decisions. If this is not the case the examination is not necessary.

➕ Remember to consider the patient's GBS status when making decisions about induction of labour with SROM.

References:
NICE Guideline CG190- Intrapartum Care for Healthy Women and Babies

3.18 Hypertension (2)

Scenario

A 25-year-old nulliparous woman is referred to you by her community midwife at 26 weeks gestation with a blood pressure of 155/95 mmHg. Her booking blood pressure was 125/85. Her urine dipstick is NAD. She is complaining of dizziness, and occasional headaches. Her observations are otherwise normal. You have been asked to come and review her in antenatal clinic.

What is your differential diagnosis?

Anxiety
Pregnancy-induced hypertension (PIH)
Chronic hypertension
Pre-eclampsia
The most common cause of high blood pressure in pregnancy is anxiety or stress, with many women being nervous when attending their antenatal appointments. It is therefore important to recheck the blood pressure, to ensure this is not the case.

How would you acutely manage this patient?

This patient should be managed using the ABCDE approach. After establishing haemodynamic stability, a full history and examination should then be completed.

Airway: Ensure the airway is patent and protected. Pregnant women with hypertension could develop eclampsia and lose their ability to maintain their airway.

Breathing: Respiratory rate is important in ruling out anxiety.

Circulation: Assess the blood pressure and re-check if required. Make sure to check this both electronically and manually. Measure the heart rate. Take bloods for FBC, U+Es, LFT, transaminases, and uric acid if indicated by the severity of hypertension. In severe hypertension, place a large bore cannula.

Disability: Use the AVPU/GCS scoring system to assess neurological status. Seizures and cerebrovascular events are a serious risk of hypertension in pregnancy.

Exposure: Check for peripheral oedema and consider checking reflexes.

What investigation would aid your diagnosis?

Confirm hypertension: A diagnosis of hypertension can be established with either a single reading of diastolic blood pressure of 110 mmHg, or two read-

CLINICAL

ings of 140/90 mmHg 4 hours apart. It is important to establish the severity of hypertension when considering further investigations.

Urine sample: A urine sample will be required for both dipstick, and urinary protein:creatinine ratio in order to quantify the proteinuria.

Serum blood samples:
In mild hypertension: Routine antenatal care bloods only
In moderate and severe hypertension: FBC, with platelets, U+Es, transaminases, bilirubin and uric acid.

What is the definition of Pregnancy-Induced Hypertension?

New hypertension, developing after 20 weeks, with no significant proteinuria.

What defines significant proteinuria?

A urine protein:creatinine ratio of greater than 30 mg/mmol.

What risk factors need to be considered for additional assessment and follow-up?

Age ≥ 40 years
Nulliparity
Multiple pregnancy
Personal history of pregnancy-induced hypertension, or pre-eclampsia
Family history of pregnancy-induced hypertension, or pre-eclampsia
A pregnancy interval ≥ 10 years
BMI ≥ 35 kg/m2
Gestational age at presentation
Pre-existing vascular or renal disease

What follow-up is required in pregnancy-induced hypertension in the antenatal period?

Mild hypertension: Blood pressure monitoring no more than once a week, test for proteinuria using automated reagent-strip reading device or urinary protein:creatinine ratio at each visit, and no further blood tests unless indicated by escalation in hypertension, or development of proteinuria. Women with pregnancy-induced hypertension presenting before 32 weeks, or with a high risk profile of developing pre-eclampsia, blood pressure and urine tests should be performed twice weekly.

Moderate hypertension: Blood pressure monitoring at least twice a week, test for proteinuria using automated reagent-strip reading device or urinary protein:creatinine ratio at each visit, and no further blood tests unless indicated by escalation in hypertension, or development of proteinuria.

Severe hypertension: Admission to hospital until blood pressure is below 159/109, blood pressure monitoring at least four times a day, test for proteinuria using automated reagent-strip reading device or urinary protein:creatinine ratio daily, and blood test required weekly. After effective control of the hypertension, and subsequent discharge from hospital, measure blood pressure and test urine twice weekly, and continue blood tests weekly.

CLINICAL

What is the treatment of pregnancy-induced hypertension?

Antihypertensive treatment: antihypertensive treatment is required in moderate and severe pregnancy-induced hypertension, with the latter requiring hospital admission for close monitoring. The aim is to maintain diastolic blood pressure between 80-100 mmHg, and systolic blood pressure less than 150 mmHg. First-line therapy is oral labetalol. After individual side-effects profiles have been considered alternative antihypertensive can be offered, including methyldopa and nifedipine.

Hospital admission for bed rest is not recommended, and should not be offered, as a treatment of pregnancy-induced hypertension.

Timing of birth: If the woman has pregnancy-induced hypertension with a blood pressure of less than 160/110, with or without treatment, do not offer birth before 37 weeks gestation. Timing of birth, along with maternal and fetal indications should be agreed upon with the woman if after 37 weeks gestation. If the woman has refractory severe pregnancy-induced hypertension, offer birth post completion of a corticosteroid course.

SUMMARY

Pregnancy-induced hypertension is defined as new hypertension with no significant proteinuria, after 20 weeks gestation. Therefore, if hypertension is noted before this, the diagnosis is chronic hypertension, not pregnancy-induced hypertension.

The most common cause of a high blood pressure in pregnant women is anxiety, or stress. It is therefore important to re-check the blood pressure a few hours later, and to ask for this information in your history. If hypertension is confirmed, ensure you consider the risk factors of developing pre-eclampsia, in addition to the investigation results, when deciding on the frequency of monitoring. Oral labetalol is the first line therapy, if treatment is required, but make sure to consider the patient's medical history, and allergies, when deciding upon antihypertensive treatment. Ensure a care plan is sent to the GP on discharging postnatal women with pregnancy-induced hypertension.

TOP TIPS

 Remember to confirm hypertension prior to diagnosis. Many patients will be hypertensive due to anxiety.

 Do not forget to consider risk factors of developing pre-eclampsia, in conjunction with the severity of hypertension, when deciding on frequency of monitoring during the antenatal period.

References:
National Collaborating Centre for Women's and Children's Health (UK). Hypertension in Pregnancy: The Management of Hypertensive Disorders During Pregnancy. London: RCOG Press; 2010 Aug. (NICE Clinical Guidelines, No. 107.)

3.19 Post-Partum Haemorrhage (PPH) (2)

Scenario

You are the ST1 on call and are asked to review an unwell postnatal admission. The patient is 6 days post normal vaginal delivery and presents feeling unwell and with fresh PV bleeding and clots.

What is your differential diagnosis?

This scenario is for secondary post-partum haemorrhage which is defined as bleeding between 24 hours and 12 weeks post delivery. The two most common causes are endometritis and retained products of conception.

Symptoms include: fever, abdominal pain, offensive lochia, dyspareunia, dysuria and general malaise.
Risk factors include: extended labour, difficult third stage and ragged placental membranes. There may be fever, rigors, tachycardia, suprapubic tenderness and tender adnexae. Elevated fundus abdominal palpation which classically feels 'boggy' with RPOC.

How would you acutely manage this patient?

Airway and Breathing: a high concentration of oxygen (10–15 litres/minute) via a facemask should be administered, regardless maternal oxygen concentration. If the airway is compromised owing to impaired conscious level, anaesthetic assistance should be sought urgently.

Circulation: establish two large bore cannulae; 20 ml blood sample should be taken and sent. Transfuse blood as soon as possible if rapid losses occurring. Warmed IV fluids
Uterotonics as medical management of excessive bleeding.

Disability: monitor conscious level using AVPU or GCS scoring system

Exposure: examine to assess tone of uterus and exclude other sources of bleeding. Keep the woman warm using appropriate available measures. Pass speculum to exclude lacerations of cervix and lower genital tract as well as possible clots in the cervical os.

For Endometritis: the sepsis 6 should be performed ASAP: blood cultures, IV antibiotics (within the hour), high flow O2, IV fluids, serum lactate, catheterise.

If RPOC are suspected, ERPC with antibiotic cover may well be necessary. The uterus is at high risk of perforation during this time.

What investigation would aid your diagnosis

High and low vaginal swabs: to assess for infection

Blood cultures if pyrexial
Serum lactate: as per sepsis 6 guidance
Full blood count, C-reactive protein - to assess for infection
MSU
Pelvic US may help to exclude the presence of RPOC, although the appearance of the uterus soon after delivery may be unreliable.

What are the risk factors for Secondary PPH?

- Prolonged rupture of membranes
- Severe meconium staining in liquor
- Extended labour with multiple examinations
- Manual removal of placenta
- Maternal anaemia
- Prolonged surgery
- Internal fetal monitoring
- General anaesthetic

What are some clinical signs of sepsis?

- Fever
- Rigors
- Sustained tachycardia
- Raised respiratory rate
- Tender boggy uterus
- Adnexal tenderness
- Offensive vaginal discharge or lochia

Can you name any rarer causes of secondary post-partum haemorrhage?

- Puerperal inversion of the uterus
- Uterine polyp or fibroid
- Undiagnosed cervical carcinoma
- Choriocarcinoma

Give some of the complications of major haemorrhage postpartum

- Hypovolaemic shock
- Disseminated intravascular coagulation
- Renal and liver failure
- ARDS
- Death

Can you name the 'sepsis 6'?

Give 3: IV antibiotics, oxygen, IV fluids
Take 3: Blood cultures, lactate, catheterise

What are some of the risks and complications of ERPC post-partum?

Increased risk of uterine perforation
Infection
Further bleeding
Intrauterine adhesions or Asherman's syndrome

What are the common organisms causing sepsis in the puerperium, including hospital- acquired infection?

GAS, also known as Streptococcus pyogenes.
Escherichia coli
Staphylococcus aureus
Streptococcus pneumonia
Meticillin-resistant S. aureus (MRSA), Clostridium septicum and Morganella morganii.

SUMMARY

Secondary postpartum haemorrhage is defined as abnormal bleeding from 24 hours after delivery. It is usually due to infection (endometritis) or retained products of conception. Resuscitation should proceed as per ABCDE approach with particular emphasis on the sepsis 6 criteria and administration of IV antibiotics within the hour if signs of infection are present. Uterotonics are used to medically manage excessive bleeding. If RPOC present ERPC is the mainstay of surgical management. This is high risk in the postpartum period as the uterus is particularly friable and very easy to perforate.

CLINICAL

TOP TIPS

➕ The key to this scenario is to show the panel you are aware the two most common causes of delayed bleeding post-partum are infection and retained products.

➕ Keep a structured approach to resuscitation and management including ABCDE and sepsis 6.

3.20 Fetal Distress (2)

Scenario

A 23-year-old patient in her first pregnancy with known DCDA twins and polyhydramnios presents to the antenatal assessment unit at 35/40 for a routine CTG check. On arrival the patient's CTG was initially normal, but during the assessment her membranes rupture spontaneously and now there are signs of fetal distress on the CTG with atypical decelerations and a rising baseline. You are walking past and are asked to review her by one of the midwives who appears very concerned. The midwife informs you that she thinks the first twin is breech.

What is your differential diagnosis

CTG concerns:
- Fetal distress/hypoxia
- Cord compression and/or umbilical cord prolapse/vasospasm

Acute causes of fetal distress on a CTG include:

- Placental abruption
- Umbilical cord prolapse *(most likely in this scenario)*
- Uterine hyperstimulation *(unlikely in this cord considering she has not had pros tin or syntocinon)*
- Uterus rupture *(unlikely in a patient who has not had a previous caesarean section, although not impossible)*

Other causes to consider:

- Pre-term labour
- Chorioamnionitis

In this case cord prolapse is very likely given that the patient has multiple risk factors for it. This included ruptured membranes, twin pregnancy, breech presentation and polyhydramnios.

How would you acutely manage this patient?

In the case of a pathological CTG the emergency protocol should be instigated immediately. Call for help; request an emergency call for the obstetric and neonatal team. Supply the patient with high flow oxygen (15L) via a non-rebreathe mask, this will reduce the effects of fetal hypoxia in the short term. Request that two large bore IV cannulas be sited (and bloods taken) whilst assessing the patient for delivery.

It is important to consider a cord prolapse in the case immediately and therefore a quick ABCD assessment of the woman should be followed by an immediate vaginal examination. If the cord is palpable then the fetal head should be lifted away from the cord to prevent its compression. The hand needs to remain here until delivery of the fetus. The cord should be kept in the vagina or higher in

CLINICAL

the genital tract to keep it warm and you should try not to palpate it as this can cause spasm. It can help to insert a catheter to lift the baby's head away from the cord. It is also recommended that the woman positions herself on all 4s and elevates her bottom. If the patient is fully dilated an instrumental delivery may be achievable, otherwise a category one caesarean section is required. Theatre teams should be notified immediately and verbal consent for category 1 section is acceptable. The baby needs to be delivered quickly and cord gases upon delivery should be taken.

In the case of umbilical cord prolapse in the community, urgent hospital transfer should be sought. In the interim tocolytics, bladder filling and maternal positioning as suggested before need to be commenced. Again the cord should not be handled in order to prevent vasospasm. If there is a lot of cord hanging outside the vagina this should be kept warm and gently placed in the vagina if possible.

At all times it is important to communicate effectively with the patient, relatives and the obstetric and neonatal teams; as well as document events clearly.

What investigation would aid your diagnosis

Umbilical cord prolapse is a clinical diagnosis usually based on examination findings. However were this not the case, a pathological CTG may warrant fetal blood sampling dependent on the clinical picture. A result greater than or equal to pH 7.25 is normal and should be repeated in one hour if the CTG remains pathological, between 7.21 and 7.24 is borderline and should be repeated in thirty minutes. A result less than or equal to 7.20 is abnormal and should be considered for delivery.

What is the definition of umbilical cord prolapse?

Umbilical cord decent through the cervix either alongside occult or past overt the presenting part in the presence of ruptured membranes

How common is umbilical cord prolapse?

This condition has an incidence in the UK of approximately 0.1-0.6% and 1% in breech presentations.

What are the antenatal risk factors for umbilical cord prolapse?
- Breech presentation
- Unstable lie
- Oblique/transverse lie
- Polyhydramnios
- External cephalic version
- Expectant management of premature rupture of membranes
- Previous cord prolapse
- Multiple pregnancy

CLINICAL

What are the intrapartum risk factors for umbilical cord prolapse?

- Amniotomy *(especially with a high presenting part)*
- Prematurity and low fetal weight
- Breech presentation
- Internal podalic version
- Second twin
- Disimpaction of fetal head during rotational assisted delivery
- Fetal scalp electrode application

How should cord prolapse be managed at the threshold of viability?

The threshold of viability is considered between 23/40 and 24+6/40. Expectant management should be discussed. There is no evidence to support cord replacement if this occurs at or before the threshold and women should have the option of pregnancy continuation or termination under consultant led care.

SUMMARY

Cord prolapse most commonly occurs by slipping below the presenting part following rupture of membranes leading to compression of the cord and compromise of the fetal blood supply. Continuous CTG monitoring is essential. This is more likely when the presenting part is poorly applied to the cervix. This is considered an obstetric emergency and necessitates immediate delivery of the fetus by the quickest and safest route possible. Should membranes be intact, the cord may still prolapse below the presenting part, this is referred to as cord/funic presentation.

TOP TIPS

 This is an obstetric emergency – clearly state this once identified. When managing emergency situations it is easy to neglect focus on communication with both the patient and partner/relatives, it is important to inform them of events as they happen and include them in the debrief. Visualisation of a prolapsed cord can be a very tempting prospect – do not handle the cord or try to replace it.

References:
PROMPT Course Handbook

4 COMMUNICATION

COMMUNICATION

4.1 Angry Relative

Scenario

You are the SHO on call and have been asked to speak to Mr Morton on the postnatal ward. You know that Mrs Morton has successfully given birth to a live male baby via a planned elective caesarean section earlier that morning, followed by a tubal ligation procedure. You have washed your hands and introduced yourself. Please talk to Mr Morton and elicit his concerns.

How would you begin?

You: "Hello Mr Morton, my name is Dr X and I am one of the team members in obstetrics and gynaecology. First of all, many congratulations on the birth of your son. I have come to see if I can answer any of your questions, if you had any?"

66 **Relative:** *[angrily] "Yes. I am very angry and I would like to make a complaint against the obstetric team"*

Continue to gather information, let the patient speak and be sympathetic.

You: "I am sorry you are feeling like this Mr Morton. Is there anything I can do to help?"

66 **Relative:** *"It's probably too late for that now, isn't it? My wife has just had a caesarean section and we've had a baby boy, which I was obviously thrilled about. But I have just been told by my wife that during the caesarean section the team have sterilised her. I know that this was her request but I'm lost for words by this decision. "*

You: "I'm very sorry that you have just been told about this Mr Morton. Have you discussed this with your wife and her obstetric team?"

66 **Relative:** *"Yes, but I feel they have just fobbed me off."*

You: "Could you tell me what you have already been told?"

66 **Relative:** *"Just that it means that we can't have anymore children."*

You: "The procedure your wife has had is called tubal ligation, and it does stop a woman from getting pregnant. It is considered a permanent method of contraception. I can understand that you must be going through a number of feelings at the moment, but is there anything in particular about this situation that is making you feel like this?"

66 Relative: *"Well, other than the fact that I won't be a father again, I just can't believe she made a decision like this without discussing it with me first, and that the team actually agreed to do such a major procedure without my consent. What about if I wanted more children, do you not need to speak to us both before that? What if something had happened to her?"*

You: "I want to assure you that your wife is doing very well after the operation and there were no issues during the procedure. Perhaps when you feel you are ready Mr Morton, do you feel it may help to speak to your wife about how you are feeling?"

66 Relative: *"Maybe, but I'm too angry to speak to her at the moment. Honestly, I'm not even angry at her. I'm angrier with her obstetrician, how could he have not included me in the decision as big as sterilisation? A C-section is major enough!"*

You: "All your concerns are very understandable Mr Morton. As doctors we have our patient's best interests at heart, and would never have done anything that we felt would endanger your wife, especially after a C-section, which you rightly said is a major procedure in itself. Because it was your wife's decision to undergo tubal ligation, as the obstetric team taking care of her we had to respect that, and we are bound to confidentiality among patients. I a however very sorry that it has distressed you."

66 Relative: *"I understand it is her decision. I feel like I have been left in the dark. I feel betrayed, to be honest with you."*

You: "I can understand how you are feeling Mr Morton, but as doctors we are bound by our confidentiality to our patients, and in this case the decision to let you know about the procedure was not ours to make. Would it be helpful if I talked through the procedure with you so you can understand it better?"

66 Relative: *"I guess so, I don't even know what they've done to her…"*

You: "Please interrupt me at any point if a question comes up. As you are aware, she has had a caesarean section. After your baby was delivered, the surgeon would have performed the tubal ligation. It's a simple procedure lasting a few minutes which involves tying the fallopian tubes closed, which means the woman's eggs can no longer be fertilised by her partner's sperm through sexual intercourse."

66 Relative: *"Oh okay, I thought it was extensive surgery."*

What will you ask next?

You: "Could you tell me if there is anything else in particular that is making you feel anxious?"

66 Relative: *"I feel like that is our family finished now."* [sniffling]

You: "I can see that this is an emotional time for you Mr Morton. Is there anything else I can do for you?"

66 Relative: *"No…"* [continues to sniffle]

You: "Let me pass you a tissue, sometimes it can help to talk to people that have been through a similar situation, do you think that would help?"

66 Relative: *"I'm not much of a big talker. I just wish my wife could have talked to me about how she felt about this before she went ahead with the procedure. Then at least, I could have understood her side of it."*

You: "If you think it would help, I could organise for you to talk with your wife in a quiet room on the ward away from the busy patient bay she is in. It would give you the opportunity to ask all the questions you need to, in privacy."

66 Relative: *"Yes, that would help me. I would like to speak to her."*

You: "I will arrange for that to happen this afternoon when she is feeling stronger. Does that work for you?"

66 Relative: *"Yes that sounds fine. Thank you."*

What else would you ask?

You: "I know there are lots of factors making you feel angry and anxious. Would it be helpful if I answered any other questions you may have about tubal ligation?"

66 Relative: *"Well I know that you said this is a form of permanent contraception and we already have 3 children. But is there any chance she could get pregnant again?"*

You: "Tubal ligation is a method to stop women getting pregnant, and we only advise it when women are sure they do not want further children. But as with any form of contraception, there is still a small chance of getting pregnant, and we usually say 1 in 200 women who have undergone tubal ligation will become pregnant. However, unfortunately there is a chance that if you do fall pregnant, the pregnancy may develop outside the womb in the fallopian tube, and this is what we call an ectopic pregnancy."

66 Relative: *"That doesn't sound right. If after talking to my wife, we decide we do still want to continue trying for a family, can't we just get rid of the ligation of the tubes?"*

COMMUNICATION

You: "That's a good question. When we counsel women for sterilisation, we emphasize that sterilisation operations are meant to be permanent, and this is because the chances of an operation to reverse it being successful are low."

66 **Relative:** *"That's a lot to think about."*

You: "I know that's a lot to take in in one go. I will give you a leaflet that will break down the information I've given you. Also, if you think it may be helpful I can ask one of my senior colleagues, registrars or consultant who have more experience in this area to speak to you, and they will be able to address any new concerns or questions you may have."

66 **Relative:** *"I think that would help me and my wife."*

You: "I will ask them. Is there anything else that is concerning you that I can run by them?"

66 **Relative:** *"No, I think I was just angry at not being involved in the decision and not knowing what my wife had been through."*

You: "I hope I have been able to address some of your concerns Mr Morton."

66 **Relative:** *"Yes, I feel a lot calmer now."*

How would you close the consultation?

You: "I am glad you have voiced your concerns and hopefully I have managed to address some of them. I will ask a senior doctor to come and speak to you about tubal ligation. If you write down any new concerns, then we can answer those for you. I understand you initially wanted to make a complaint against the team, I would be happy to point you in the direction of the Patient Advice and Liason Service if you still feel this is what you would like to do. I will also organise a quiet space for you to talk to your wife."

SUMMARY

"I can understand your anger at not being involved in the decision making process for the tubal ligation, and the anxiety at not knowing what it involved. I hope I have addressed some of those concerns. I will ask my senior colleague to come to talk to you about the situation, and I will organise for you to talk to your wife in a quiet setting where you won't be disturbed. We are here to answer all your questions and to make sure your wife is well looked after."

COMMUNICATION

Actor Brief

Mr Morton is 46-year-old plumber who is angry that his wife has undergone tubal ligation at the end of her planned caesarean section and that he was not consulted or even aware of the decision until after the procedure. He is initially angry at his wife and the obstetric team for not additionally gaining his consent for the procedure, but as you delve deeper it seems one of the main issues is that he was actually worried that his wife had undergone 'an extensive procedure' in addition to the caesarean section. He has asked to speak to a member of the team about the situation.

Special Instructions: The actor is initially very aggressive when talking about the tubal ligation. If the candidate becomes defensive and keeps emphasising confidentially this will offend the actor further, making them angrier and escalating the situation further. The pivotal turning points are when the candidate offers to organise talks between him and his wife and realises that the deeper underlying issue is the actor's concern for his wife's health.

TOP TIPS

➕ When dealing with angry patients and/or their relatives, it is important to get to the core of what has led them to be angry, as otherwise you cannot calm them down. I find a good way of dealing with angry patients is to show them that you understand what they are going through and that you are not against them, but that you want to work with them in finding appropriate solutions.

➕ I think one of the most important things to have an understanding about here is confidentiality; it was Mr Morton's wife's decision whether she wanted him to know about the tubal ligation, not the doctor's decision. This must be emphasised clearly and confidently.

➕ If the actor gets to the stage where they are asking you about vasectomies, it may be an indication that you are performing well in the station; you have soothed their anger and have resolved/are working towards resolving the issues and he is now challenging you further.

COMMUNICATION

4.2 | Anxious Patient

Scenario

Susan is a 46-year-old diabetic patient admitted under the care of the gynaecology team for elective open laparotomy for the removal of a large fibroid uterus. The procedure is scheduled as an afternoon case but she has arrived on the ward this morning to have an insulin sliding scale set up pre-procedure. As the gynaecology SHO, you are called by the nurses to speak to Susan as her nurse reports she appears visibly distressed and is saying she no longer wants to go through with the procedure.

How would you begin the consultation?

You: "Hello Susan, my name is Dr X, I'm one of the doctors on the gynaecology team. I just came to check how you are this morning; your nurse mentioned you were upset. Is there anything I can help you with?"

❝ Patient: *[Visibly distressed] "I'm sorry, I'm just being silly, I just feel so overwhelmed by the whole thing and don't know if I can go through with it."*

What would you ask next?

You: [Comes to sit down next to patient] "Do you mean the surgery?"

❝ Patient: *[Nods, on the verge of tears] "I just feel so silly for getting so upset but I honestly don't feel like I can have the surgery, I'm sorry."*

You: "There's absolutely nothing to feel silly about, it's completely natural to feel nervous before an operation, most people do, especially if they haven't had surgery before. No-one will make you have the operation if you don't want it but you're in very safe hands. Do you think it might help if we had a chat about it?"

❝ Patient: *"I've already had it explained to me but I just feel so overwhelmed by it all …"*

You: "That's completely understandable; it's a lot to take in. Maybe you'd like to tell me if there's anything in particular about the operation that's worrying you and I can try and put some of your fears to rest?"

❝ Patient: *"I just…I know it sounds overly dramatic but I'm just so scared about being put to sleep and not waking up again. And you hear horror stories of people waking up in the middle of an operation and no-one knows about it. When I found out I was going to need a hysterectomy I looked it up online and thought I was going to have it done keyhole but then I got told it was going to be through an open cut and it just sounds*

COMMUNICATION

like such a huge thing to have done. I know plenty of people have operations but I'm anxious at the best of times and I just don't need this at the moment" [starts crying].

You: [Pass patient a tissue] "I completely understand what you're saying and it's absolutely normal to be nervous. And you're right, a lot of the time we can do a hysterectomy by keyhole surgery but the reason you're having what we call a 'laparotomy' which is an open procedure is because unfortunately you've got quite a few large fibroids and your womb is too large to take out by the very small incisions we use in keyhole surgery. So it is a bigger procedure, but it's one that is still performed commonly and we'll be monitoring you at all times during surgery to check you're OK."

66 Patient: *"But surely if it's such a big operation I'm going to lose so much blood?"*

You: "Well, it's normal and expected that patients do have some blood loss during an operation but there's no reason that you'll lose so much that it becomes unsafe. If you remember when you came to the pre-assessment clinic we did tests then to check if you were healthy enough for the operation and one of those was to check that your blood levels weren't too low that your body wouldn't cope with some blood loss. And even if there was unexpected extra bleeding we make provisions for that and can give you replacement blood quickly if you need it. Is there anything else about the surgery you're particularly worried about?"

What would you ask next?

66 Patient: *"I'm sorry, I don't want you to think I don't trust the doctors, it's just overwhelming and... this is going to sound so stupid and I know it sounds irrational because it's not like I even want any more children but I've read about women who've had hysterectomies who've said they felt like they lost their femininity when their womb was taken away. It's something that defines you as a woman and I just feel like having it removed is going to really affect me."*

You: "It doesn't irrational at all, that's something that a lot of women are worried about before a hysterectomy and some of them do say they feel like that after the operation, at least for a little while. But far more women who were in your position and have their fibroids taken away are just so glad to be free from the symptoms they've been causing and that's something to look forward to."

66 Patient: *"I know, I know it makes sense to have it done, it's just come at such a bad time, I really don't have time to be in hospital, my mum isn't very well at the moment and I need to be looking after her. And I'm self-employed and going to be losing work whilst I'm in hospital and I just can't afford that. The doctor I saw previously said I was going to have* *to stay in for the procedure but is that really necessary? It's stressful enough having the operation without worrying about everything else falling apart whilst I'm in here."*

You: "I'm sorry to hear about your mum and I can completely appreciate why you'd want to get out of hospital as soon as possible. But as we've talked about, the surgery is a bit more invasive than the keyhole so we really would like to keep an eye on you for a few days just to check that everything is going OK. It'd be much better for you and your family if we can be sure you're well and there aren't any complications rather than you having to come back in if there are problems."

The patient has some specific questions for you

❝ Patient: *"I thought you said it was a safe procedure? Why would there be any problems if it's safe?"*

You: "It is a safe procedure compared to lots of other operations that people have but any kind of surgery carries a risk of complications and we always have to bear those in mind."

❝ Patient: *"What complications?"*

You: "Well, anyone has an operation we like to keep an eye on the site where the incision was made to check it's healing well, which is especially important in your case because you have diabetes as this can sometimes affect wound healing. You also won't feel like moving around as much as usual for a few days because of the cut we make and that's another reason to stay in hospital; if you're here we can give you a medicine to keep your blood thin to prevent blood clots which are more likely to happen if you aren't moving around as much as usual. It's also important to make sure you've got an adequate amount of painkiller medicines which sometimes have to be given through a drip. I know it's frustrating and no-one likes having to stay in hospital but it really is for the best. It'll only be for a few days and the sooner we get you better the sooner you can go home."

❝ Patient: *"I just wish I could have avoided this. I know it's not cancer or anything and people have worse things happen to them but it's still got me so worried."*

You: "I completely understand and it's normal to be nervous. But no-one will make you have the procedure if you don't want to; you can change your mind. Do you still want to go ahead?"

❝ Patient: *[Shakes head] "Yes, yes I know I need to have it done, I'm just nervous. "*

COMMUNICATION

You: "Is there anything else in particular about the surgery that you're worried about?"

> **Patient:** *"There's nothing specific at the moment but I'm sure I'll have lots of questions after you've left."*

How would you close the consultation?

You: "That's no problem, I will be around on the ward all day so if you think of anything specific I can come back and we can talk through things some more. The anaesthetist, who is the doctor who will be putting you to sleep and monitoring you during the operation, will also be coming to check on you later today before the operation so you can ask anything you think of then as well. I know it's scary but you're in safe hands and you'll be well looked after."

The patient has a few further questions

> **Patient:** *[Smiles slightly] "Yes thanks. I just wish I could have avoided this, how did the fibroids even get there in the first place?"*

You: "They're extremely common so you're by no means alone, about three quarters of women will develop them at some point. They are what we call 'benign' which basically means non-cancerous tumours which develop from the muscle in the wall of the womb."

> **Patient:** *"So it's nothing in particular I did?"*

You: "Well, we're not exactly sure why fibroids develop in some people and not others but like a lot of things it seems to be a combination of various factors. For example, we know they become more frequent as women get older until before the menopause. Plus women who are exposed to more oestrogen, for example those who started their periods at a young age or have a late menopause, are more likely to develop them, as are obese women. They're also much more common in Afro-Caribbean women because your genes also have an influence on whether you develop them."

> **Patient:** *"But if they're in the genes does that mean that my daughter will develop them as well?"*

You: "Not necessarily. The risk of developing fibroids does seem to be between two and three times higher if you have a close relative with fibroids, for example a mother, but they are extremely common regardless and many women who develop fibroids don't have family members who have had them. Also, the majority of women who do develop them don't realise they're there because they don't cause bothersome symptoms."

> **Patient:** *"So if I have the surgery today will that be the end of my symptoms?"*

COMMUNICATION

You: "The symptoms caused by your fibroids, yes. It will be uncomfortable after the surgery but then the pain will go and there will be no heavy periods."

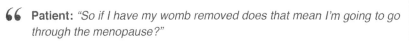 **Patient:** *"So if I have my womb removed does that mean I'm going to go through the menopause?"*

You: "Well as we've mentioned you won't have periods anymore. But a lot of the symptoms of the menopause such as the hot flushes, night sweats and vaginal dryness are actually controlled by hormones produced by your ovaries and because you're not having your ovaries removed you won't have these symptoms."

 Patient: *[Smiles] "That's reassuring, thanks."*

SUMMARY

'I really hope I've answered some of your questions and helped put your mind at rest at least a little. It sounds like you're having a really tough time at the moment and it's completely normal to be nervous before an operation. But you're in safe hands and the thing to focus on is how much better you'll feel after your surgery. I'm around on the ward today so as I've mentioned, any further questions just let me know and we can talk through things some more."

 Actor Brief

Your character's name is Susan, a 46 year old lady who has been admitted to hospital today for a planned hysterectomy to remove her uterus which contains several large fibroids. As someone who suffers from chronic anxiety and has a family to look after you are extremely nervous having such a large operation and taking time out to recover from it afterwards.

Presenting complaint:
The hysterectomy is being performed because your uterus contains large fibroids which are causing significant pain and heavy and prolonged menstrual bleeding, both of which are having a detrimental impact on your quality of life. The gynaecology consultant has already explained to you the procedure is going to be an open laparotomy, which means removing the uterus via an incision in the abdomen.

COMMUNICATION

Ideas, concerns, expectations

- You have never had surgery before and are terrified at the prospect of doing so. You are particularly worried about being 'put to sleep' and not waking up from the anaesthetic, and about losing too much blood during the operation and dying on the table.
- You are worried about feeling less feminine after your uterus is removed, although you feel silly admitting that this is one of your biggest concerns.

TOP TIPS

 As with any patient-doctor encounter the key to this consultation is developing a rapport with the patient such that she feels able to tell you specifically why she is so distressed. The patient in this scenario is an anxious lady who has personal insight and becomes frustrated with her tendency to 'think the worst', and as such the key to alleviating her worries is to reassure her that her concerns are not irrational, that it is normal to have questions and anxieties before surgery and they are not something she needs to apologise for. Your role here is to respond to these concerns with clear explanations and a non-judgemental attitude. This is specifically relevant when the patient discusses her worry that she will feel 'less feminine' post-procedure. This is something that a lot of women worry about, even if they have completed their families, and is not something to belittle.

 An appreciation for the bigger picture in this patient's case is essential. Both she and you as the doctor can appreciate that surgery is in her best interests but this lady has dependents to look after who she tends to put first. Empathising with her situation and emphasising that by putting herself first in the short-term she will be better placed to look after her family is a positive approach in this scenario.

4.3   Breaking Bad News (1)

Scenario

You are an SHO working in the early pregnancy assessment unit and have been asked to counsel Mrs Keen regarding her increased risk of her next pregnancy for trisomy 21. Mrs Keen is 44 years old and has had three children 18 years ago. She is now 12/40 gestation.

You have washed your hands, correctly identified Mrs Keen and introduced yourself. Please proceed to discuss her high risk and suggest a management plan.

How would you begin?

You: "Hello my name is Dr X. I am one of the obstetrics and gynaecology doctors. Thank you for coming along this afternoon. I have come to discuss any questions you may have. What would you like to discuss with me today?"

❝ Patient: *"I think I've just come for a general check-up for my pregnancy after my screening tests. I'm not too sure why I've had to see a doctor instead of a midwife. I have had pregnancies in the past so I know how it all works you see."*

You: "I see. Please can you tell me a little more about your previous pregnancies?"

❝ Patient: *"Well I've had three pregnancies, my eldest is 18 and the other two 16 and 14. My partner and I thought we wouldn't have any further children and this pregnancy has come as quite a surprise to us. My previous pregnancies were fine, I didn't see a doctor for any of them and they were all born normally without any problems. My husband and I are so lucky."*

You: "And do you mind telling me what's happened to you so far in this pregnancy?"

❝ Patient: *"My pregnancy so far has been absolutely fine. I've had my dating scan and a blood test so far. I think everyone is just so cautious these days! The midwife told me some of the tests were screening for conditions the baby could have, like Down's Syndrome, but as I said, my husband and I have been so lucky!"*

You: "I think today it is important we discuss these screening tests today. Has anyone discussed the results of these screening tests with you yet?"

COMMUNICATION

66 Patient: *"The midwife said the majority of them were fine but I might need to discuss my Downs Syndrome result with a doctor. I assumed they would be fine. Do you have any information about them?"*

You: "Yes I do. [Pause] I think it is important to clarify, however, that these screening tests only give us a likelihood of your baby having Down's syndrome, so results are not for certain and there are further tests we can do to get definitive answers. [Pause]. We divide the likelihood into low risk and high risk. High risk is between having a 1 in 2 chance to a 1 in 150 chance of having a baby with Down's syndrome. [Pause]. In light of the results from your screening test, your likelihood is 1 in 30 chance. Do you understand what this means?"

66 Patient: *"So my baby might have Down's syndrome?"*

You: "Yes Mrs Keen, there is an increased chance you baby may. This screening test does not tell us for certain. If you wished, we could do a further test which would give us a definitive result whether the baby has Down's syndrome."

What will you ask next?

You: "What are your thoughts regarding this information Mrs Keen?"

66 Patient: *[starts to cry].*

You: "I can appreciate this is a shock to you. I am sorry to see you're so upset. Is there anything in particular regarding this you are concerned about which we haven't covered?"

66 Patient: *"I was already so worried about a baby and three teenagers at home, and now... I just don't know how I will cope... I am worried this is my fault. Is it because of something I have done? How did the tests know that I have an increased risk?"*

You: "No, it is not your fault. There is no evidence that actions before pregnancy or during pregnancy cause Down's syndrome. It occurs because of an error in the baby's genetic material.
Your risk is calculated from the ultrasound scan measuring the fluid behind baby's neck, it's length and a blood test showing the amount of two types of protein in your blood. Unfortunately the older you are when you are pregnant, the increased the chance are to have a baby with Down's syndrome.
Does that make sense to you? I just want to clarify again, the screening test result just gives us a likelihood, and it is not for certain."

The patient has some specific questions for you

66 Patient: *"Yes it does. I think my husband would feel the same that I need to have the further test for the baby. It is important we should know. What is it?"*

You: "The test we would do would give a definitive answer as to whether the baby has Down's syndrome. The purpose is so that you and your family can make an informed decision about your pregnancy and if you continue with the pregnancy it helps you prepare for a baby with increased needs. The test is called chorionic villus sampling."

66 **Patient:** *"How would I have it done?"*

You: "The sample of the placenta is usually taken by inserting a needle through the skin into the placenta through the tummy wall, under ultrasound guidance. A very small amount of tissue from the placenta which supplies baby with blood will be taken out and this will be tested for the baby's DNA for Down's syndrome. Getting the results will take a few days and we will be able to discuss the results with you. The test takes about ten minutes. There is a small 1% chance that the test may not work and we will need to repeat the test or do a different test."

66 **Patient:** *"Is it a safe test?"*

You: "It is a safe test, but there are some risks. The main one is that there is a 1% chance that you may miscarry after the test. The test may be uncomfortable, and you may have some light spotting for a day after and some cramping. There is also a small chance of infection, with serious infection 1 in 1000 chance."

The patient has some further questions

66 **Patient:** *"So doctor, what should I do?"*

You: "I'm afraid I can't answer that question for you. I can only give you information so you can make an informed decision on what is best for yourself. If you would like further information potential sources include; ARC service (antenatal results and choices charity), NHS choices, The Down's Syndrome association. We have some leaflets here as well for you to take home with you."

66 **Patient:** *"Doctor if my baby does actually have Down's syndrome what does that mean?"*

You: "If your baby has Down's syndrome at birth your baby might appear smaller than other babies and have reduced muscle tone so it may appear floppy. You will notice certain characteristic facial features regarding your baby's eyes, mouth, tongue and head shape and we know that babies with Down's syndrome are more likely to have learning problems."

How would you close the consultation?

"Thank you for coming in today to speak with me Mrs Keen. I appreciate this news of your baby having a high risk for Down's syndrome has come as a shock. Please take these contact numbers along with this information leaflet regarding what we have discussed today. I recommend having a read with your

COMMUNICATION

husband of the websites and support forums on the back. If you wish to come back to re-discuss anything before your next appointment, I will be very happy to do so."

SUMMARY

Understanding and managing patient expectations is key in this scenario. From the history, it should be noted that the patient's midwife had tried to convey some previous warning shots regarding her higher risk. The patient had had three previous, unremarkable pregnancies in the past and consequently felt reassured about her current pregnancy and it was difficult to break through that barrier.

 Actor Brief

You are Mrs Keen, a 44 year old woman, with three children 18, 16 and 14 years old. You are currently 12/40 weeks' gestation with an unplanned pregnancy. Your previous three pregnancies were midwife-led, with SVD with no complications. You have thus far had screening tests for conditions your baby may have. When you last saw your midwife she told you most of the tests seemed fine but you might have to discuss the Downs Syndrome result with a doctor.

TOP TIPS

➕ **Examiners are looking for:** Clear communication to identify reasons why Mrs Keen is high risk for trisomy 21 and explanation of the management of high risk for trisomy 21

➕ **Common pitfalls:** Remember the importance of sign-posting to prepare the patient for what may be unexpected news in light of her three previously normal pregnancies

➕ **Not to miss/do:** Ensure clarification of understanding and delivering information in small chunks. Highlight moving forward with this new information and negotiate a management plan with the patient where the patient has made well-informed decisions

COMMUNICATION

4.4 Confidentiality

Scenario

You are the SHO on call and you have been asked to speak to Katie Smith, a 15-year-old girl who has been found to have an ectopic pregnancy on her ultrasound scan. You have been informed that she is suitable for methotrexate therapy. She does not want her mother to know. Please talk to her about her concerns with consulting her mother. You have washed your hands and introduced yourself.

How would you begin?

You: "Hello my name is Dr X and I am one of the team members in obstetric and gynaecology. I have come to speak to you about the scan we have just done and what we can do to help you. Do you have anything you want to ask at the moment?"

❝ **Patient**: *"Ok thanks. So the last doctor told me about my baby being in the wrong place and not the womb. She said it wont continue to grow and is not viable. Do you agree? What is it?"*

How will you respond?

You: "Yes, that's correct about the baby being in the wrong place, we call it an 'ectopic pregnancy'. What has happened is that instead of the baby-sitting in the womb, the baby is sitting in the small tube that connects to your womb, which unfortunately, cannot stretch (draw picture). What that means is, as the baby grows, it can put pressure on the tube and so the tube will eventually burst. Does that make sense?"

❝ **Patient:** *"Yer I guess so. The last doctor said about having a medicine to end the pregnancy. Can you tell me about this?"*

You: "You are suitable for a medication injection called methotrexate. This needs to be given, usually as a one off dose and it stops further growth of the baby. Some patients have a little bleed and some pain with this. Some patented need a second dose. And a small percent of patients require an operation if the medication doesnt work. Some patients choose to have an operation instead of the medication. Taking the medication does involve monitoring your bloods over the course of a few days and patients must not fall pregnant for 3 months after having it."

What will you ask next?

You: "How are you feeling about it?"

COMMUNICATION

---

66 **Patient:** *"The last doctor asked me this too. I'm upset but I know that the pregnancy is dangerous to my health in the tube and it can't grow anyway where it is. Plus this wasn't planned. I don't like the idea of an operation, I heard that they take away a tube and I don't want that. What about my mum? The last Doctor said I should speak to her. Why does she need to know?"*

You: "I can see that you don't want to tell your mum. Do you mind if I ask why?"

66 **Patient:** *"I just don't want her to know. She doesn't need to know. I really don't want her involved and you can't tell her"* (patient gets angry).

You: "I understand Katie, was there something in particular that you were worried about regarding your Mums reaction should you tell her?"

66 **Patient:** *"I just can't even think about it. She'd be so annoyed. She hates my boyfriend and she has no idea I'm sleeping with him."*

How would you explore her relationship with her boyfriend to assess whether there is risk of coercion?

You: "I can see that it would be a difficult conversation to have Katie. Do you mind if I ask, why does your mum not like your boyfriend?"

66 **Patient:** *"She just thinks I can do better and doesn't like me dating someone in my class because it disrupts my studies. He's not a bad guy at all. He would be here too if he wasn't on holiday."*

You: "Ok I understand. How is everything with your boyfriend?"

66 **Patient:** *"Things are great, I love him. We celebrated our 6-month anniversary last week!"*

You: "I'm glad to hear that."

66 **Patient:** *"My Mum just doesn't need to know. And anyway, I understand what I need to do, I just need to take have this injection and then it will all be ok. She never has to know."*

You: (start assessing Gillick competence) "Katie, you are right about taking the medicines and that being the next step. But you do need to understand clearly how the medicine works, its side effects and what we would need to do, should the medicine not work. Although you are understanding what I'm saying so far, there is more I need to tell you and things that you might want the support of your mum for."

66 **Patient:** *"Ok, what do you mean? What else is there?"*

You: "Unfortunately, the medication we're giving you is not very nice to take. It does have side effects and we would need to monitor you as you take it and do regular blood tests at least two in the week following having the injection, to check your hormone level if coming down. So that would mean you'd have to come into hospital, I'm not sure if that might be difficult for you if your mum doesn't know what's going on. And just going back to what I was saying earlier, sometimes the medicine is not 100% effective unfortunately. If the medicine doesn't work, we may have to do an operation."

❝ **Patient:** *"Oh, I see, so it might not be a simple thing really."*

You: "It might not be. You might feel unwell after having it, have some bleeding or a side effect. You will need to come back for blood monitoring and it is possible that you may need a repeat injection or an operation still. How are you feeling about all this information?"

❝ **Patient:** *"I don't know, I'm just surprised. I thought you could fix things really easily and I would just walk out of here. I still don't know whether to tell my mum, I don't want to. You're not going to tell her are you?! I'm sure you're not allowed to unless I say?"*

You: "I can see that you don't want to tell your mum Katie and that you're scared. But despite being mature and understanding what I'm saying, I'm also a bit worried about how you'll go through this on your own. We do have a duty of confidentiality with our patients, but when it comes to younger people, it gets a bit complicated. Especially with you being 15, we do need to think about what's best for you emotionally and then consider whether it's best for your mum to know. But I don't want to tell her anything without your permission. I think it's best if you were to sit her down and tell her."

❝ **Patient:** *"But what if she gets angry?"*

You: "You can sit and tell her in front of me if you want, so I can help you tell her or just be there if you need me. But I'm sure she will just be worried for you and want to help you get better and help you through this situation."

❝ **Patient:** *"Ok, maybe."*

How would you close the consultation?

You: "Do you want to ask anything else at this stage? Or anything else you want to tell me?"

❝ **Patient:** *"No not really. I do want you to be there though. Is that ok?"*

You: "Of course I can be there."

The patient has a few questions for you

66 **Patient:** *"So you said how this whole confidentiality thing isn't always the case with young people like me- what does that even mean? I thought doctors aren't allowed to tell anyone anything?"*

You: "You're right in saying that doctors are meant to keep information confidential, but that strict rule is for people aged over 16. It gets a bit complicated especially when the child is younger than 16, where we need to judge as doctors, whether the patient understands the condition or treatment well enough to make a decision for themselves. We also need to encourage them to tell their parents and if not, we can only keep it confidential if we believe that the patient will cope well without the support of their parents. We just want to make sure you're well looked after and that's our priority."

66 **Patient:** *"Is surgery just a last resort option for ectopic pregnancies?"*

You: "Surgery isn't exactly the last resort, but the options depend upon how far along the pregnancy you are, if you are well or unwell and the level of the pregnancy hormone, beta hCG. So the options can be expectant, where if the hormone level is dropping and the patient is well, then we can just monitor the patient and not give any active treatment. Another option is the medical treatment, which we would like to offer you, and that's if the patient is well, the fetus is below a certain measurement and if the hormone level is in a specific range. But if the patient is very unwell or the medical treatment doesn't work, we may need to go for surgical management."

SUMMARY

"I can see how difficult this is all is for you. You have so much to think about and it seems not that many people to speak to about it and get support from. I'm sure your mum will be really helpful and supportive through all of this and especially with your boyfriend not being around, this is a big thing for you to go through on your own. I would also worry about you if I knew you were going through it alone and especially, without an adult. I'll be there while you tell your mum if you think that will help. In terms of any questions she has, I'm also very happy to answer them."

Actor Brief

You are a 15-year-old girl and are in school. You are angry at the thought of having to tell your mother about this ectopic pregnancy, but that is mainly masking your underlying fear of telling her. As the consultation progresses you come round to the idea of telling your mother but are scared and upset and would like the support of the doctor.

At first you think that there solution is simple and simply requires an injection. You are able to understand and weigh up the information.

TOP TIPS

➕ Allow the patient to express their emotions of anger towards you and then being upset and confused. There are quite a few areas to address but try not to get caught up in the details of an ectopic pregnancy as this is a communication station, so keep it simple. The facts will be asked more towards the end to push you further.

➕ Important areas to address are assessing the Gillick competence of the patient as the consultation is progressing. Also important is finding out more about the boyfriend- his age, whether he is in a position of responsibility, ascertaining whether the patient is happy in the relationship or being coerced into sleeping with him. The relationship between the patient and her father can also be explored to see if she is more comfortable talking to him than the mother.

➕ Always let the patient know you are not just there to support them medically but also emotionally and socially, hence offering to be there when the patient has the difficult conversation with her mother.

COMMUNICATION

4.5   Counselling

Scenario

You are the SHO in the antenatal clinic. Tina Smith, a 20-year-old lady has come in for her booking appointment (8 weeks pregnant). You can see from her notes that she is a smoker and is continuing to smoke in pregnancy. Please talk to Tina Smith about her smoking habits and come up with a management plan. You have washed your hands and introduced yourself.

How would you begin?

You: "Hello my name is Dr X and I am one of the team members in obstetrics and gynaecology. Congratulations on your pregnancy. I would just like to have a chat about how things are going and your general health during the pregnancy so far, if that's ok?"

66 **Patient:** *"Yes sure, things are fine."* (Patient is quite abrupt and disinterested)

Find out how much information the patient has been given and their understanding thus far

You: "That's good to hear. I see this is your first pregnancy?"

66 **Patient:** *"Yes"*

You: "How have you been feeling in yourself, have you been well?"

66 **Patient:** *"I've been fine, things have just been normal really. Haven't felt much of a difference."*

You: "Ok sure, I guess we are in early days. I was just having a look through your notes and I see that you are normally healthy and well, with no medical problems; which is great. We've also got noted down here that you smoke, is that correct?"

66 **Patient:** *"Yes, I love a fag"*

You: "Right ok. Have you been smoking since you found out you were pregnant?"

66 **Patient:** *"Yes, not given up and don't want to. It's been part of my life for 10 years now, so you can save the 'stop smoking' chat for the next person."* (Patient quite defensive)

You: "I understand it's been part of your life for a long time and so it can be very difficult to stop the habit. But has someone spoken to you about smoking in pregnancy and how that can affect your future child?"

66 **Patient:** *"My GP has tried to but she's useless, I don't listen to anything she says. I know people that smoked in pregnancy anyway, and their kids were fine."*

What will you ask next?

You: "Do you mind if I ask a bit more about how much you smoke and just how it fits into your daily routine?"

66 **Patient:** *"There's not much to say, I go through a few packs a day. I smoke when I want to."*

You: "So there's no pattern to when you smoke, for example not after a meal or when you're a bit bored..?"

66 **Patient:** *"Maybe. When I'm on my own I guess."* (Patient starts to look sad)

You: "Do you find that you're on your own often?"

66 **Patient:** *"Um kind of."* (Patient starts crying) *"My boyfriend left me 1 month ago when he found out I was pregnant"*

You: "Oh I'm so sorry, let me get you a tissue"

66 **Patient:** *"I've been smoking more since he left, I go through packs and packs. I wasn't that bad before"*

You: (comforting) "That sounds awful, I'm so sorry." (Give patient time to settle tears) "How are you feeling about this pregnancy?"

66 **Patient:** *"I really want this baby. It's all I have now."* (Patient's wiping away tears)

You: "I understand, I can see this is a really hard time for you and you are feeling quite alone. Do you think the cigarettes might be a form of coping mechanism for you at the moment, with all this stress you are going through?"

66 **Patient:** *"Definitely, I couldn't give them up right now"*

You: "Do you mind if I talk to you more about your smoking and the pregnancy?"

COMMUNICATION

66 Patient: *"Ok"*

You: "I know you said your friend's children were fine even though they smoked when pregnant, but that's not always the case unfortunately. We really do worry about smoking in pregnancy and how that can affect the unborn child."

66 Patient: *"What do you mean? I didn't think it was that big a deal, I thought it's just bad for me and my lungs and it doesn't always reach the child"*

You: "We do worry about how smoking affects you and your lungs, but the effect of tobacco can on your baby can also be really serious. In a smoking woman, the placenta can become unhealthy. The placenta is the source of oxygen and nutrients to your growing baby."

66 Patient: *"So the baby can have less nutrients, who cares, I barely have any of them in my own body anyway."*

You: "Unfortunately there are some very serious effects of a unhealthy placenta to understand. It puts you at risk of a miscarriage and stillbirth, we know that women who smoke have higher rates of preterm labour and abruption. A third of all deaths in the womb or shortly after birth are thought to be caused by smoking. It also means that your baby will have an increased risk of being born with abnormalities such as spina bifida and babies of smokers are smaller than they should be."

66 Patient: *"OK, You're really scaring me now."*

You: "I know, it is so scary and I'm sorry to tell you all these awful things that can happen. But I really want the best for you and your baby."

66 Patient: *"I know. I just can't stop smoking. I can't. It helps me feel better with everything going on."*

You: "Tina, I understand things are so difficult for you at the moment, but you really can do it. I have seen many women stop smoking and often completely give up once they're pregnant. I know that it seems to help you cope with what has happened in your life but you do need to keep yourself and the baby healthy. How would you feel about being referred to our smoking cessation clinic?"

66 Patient: *"It's just so difficult. But I also don't want anything bad to happen to the baby. You're right, I need the baby to make things better. Yes refer me, I need the support. I didn't realise how serious smoking actually was."*

How would you close the consultation?

You: "Tina, we will do everything we can to support you through this. We understand how difficult it can be but you can do it. I will refer you today to our specialised team of people to help pregnant women stop smoking and they're fantastic."

66 **Patient:** *"I'm scared and feel a bit weak, but I can try."*

You: "That's great, that's the first step; to just say that you'll try and that's sometimes that hardest step to take. With the help of this team of people and we can do everything we can to help you have a healthy little baby."

SUMMARY

"I understand there are big changes happening in your life at the moment Tina, and it is so overwhelming for you. We will do everything we can to help you give up smoking, so that not only you will be well in yourself, but also so you have a healthy baby to keep you occupied and happier. I will refer you to our smoking cessation clinic and also book you to speak with our psychologist if you would like."

 Actor Brief

You are a young 20-year-old lady who is not well kempt, not well educated and very closed off from the consultation and defensive at the beginning. It is clear you have a barrier up and are disinterested in the conversation initially, until you are probed more into your daily routine and the doctor asks if you smoke when you're bored. After the doctor has identified the reasons behind you smoking, you become very upset and start crying thinking about your loneliness, and then become more receptive in the consultation.

TOP TIPS

➕ Listen to the patient and allow them to express their emotions and pick up on any worries they may have. There is often an underlying point you need to get out of the patient. In this scenario it was that the patient has increased their cigarette intake because they are lonely after their partner left them. Once you have addressed this you can work out ways to solve the problem and the patient also becomes more receptive to your suggestions.

➕ Don't worry too much about the details of smoking in pregnancy, as this is about counselling and communication. If you are asked for facts then that is because the actor is pushing you and you are doing well.

COMMUNICATION

4.6 Explaining a Complication

Scenario

You are the SHO on call for the night shift and have been asked to speak to Mrs Brown on labour ward by your obstetric registrar as she is stuck in theatre. You know that Mrs Brown has just had a caesarean section that was complicated by a large postpartum hemorrhage (PPH) of 2000mls. You have washed your hands and introduced yourself. Please talk to Mrs Brown, explain the complication and elicit her concerns.

How would you begin?

You: "Hello my name is Dr X and I am one of the doctors on the obstetric team looking after you today. I have come to see how you are doing after the operation?"

> **Patient:** *[tired] "I'm feeling really weak and I'm in a lot of pain, I feel like I've been through the wars. I didn't realise a caesarean section would make me feel this dreadful."*

Continue to gather information, let the patient speak and be sympathetic

You: "First of all Mrs Brown, I would like to say congratulations on the birth of your baby girl, but I'm sorry that you're in pain, I'll make sure you some pain relief. Can you tell me what you have been told about the caesarean section?"

> **Patient:** *"Well they didn't tell me much during the caesarean as they were frantically doing the surgery I think. I remember someone mentioning I'd lost a bit of blood, but by that point I was just so drained I wasn't really registering what they were saying to me, to be honest."*

You: "Would it be helpful if I explained what happened during your caesarean section?"

> **Patient:** *"Yes. I guess it would be nice to know what was happening and why I'm feeling like this. "*

You: "After your baby was safely delivered, the team noticed that you were bleeding. It is normal to have some blood loss after childbirth, but unfortunately, you had actually lost quite a large volume of blood. It's what we call a postpartum haemorrhage."

> **Patient:** *[Bewildered] "I don't understand... are you saying I had a complication during my operation? Could I have died?"*

You: "Unfortunately, some people who undergo caesarean sections are at risk of developing PPH, which is a recognised complication. Yes, it can be life threatening. I am sorry that you had to go through that Mrs Brown. The important thing is that we treated it early and that you are stable now. Is there anything in particular that is causing you concern?"

66 **Patient:** *[Angry] "I just don't understand why I am only finding out about this complication now?"*

You: "Again, I would like to reiterate how sorry I am that you have had to go through this ordeal. I can understand that you must be feeling angry and confused. At the time when you started to bleed, the team were working really hard to do everything to stop the bleeding and minimise any further blood loss and complications. We would have attempted to let you know what was happening at the time, but the team felt that our priority at the time was to deal with the situation at hand promptly, and to allow you to recover sufficiently before explaining anything to you."

66 **Patient:** *[Angry] "Did the surgeon not know what he was doing? I would like to make a formal complaint if that is the case."*

You: "I assure you Mrs Brown that your surgeon was very experienced and has performed many caesarean sections. PPH is an unfortunate complication of caesarean sections and is, sometimes unavoidable. If you would still like to make a complaint, however, it is completely your right to do so and I can refer you to the Patient Advice and Liaison Service."

66 **Patient***: [Angry & teary] "Are you saying that it's my fault then?"*

You: "Mrs Brown, I want to reassure you that this is not your fault in anyway; you must not blame yourself for this. There are a number of reasons why women develop PPH and you are not alone, in fact, around 6% of births are complicated by PPH."

What will you ask next?

You: "Could you tell me if there is anything in particular that is worrying you or has upset you?"

66 **Patient***: "I just don't get why this happened to me then? I was so careful during this pregnancy. I went for all my check-ups."*

You: "I appreciate it must be very difficult to understand why this has happened, but there's nothing you could have done. You've done all the right things in this pregnancy. Would it help if I talked to you a bit more about PPH?"

COMMUNICATION

Patient: *"I guess it would. Do you think this has happened because I had a few glasses of wine early in my pregnancy? But I didn't even know I was pregnant then, honestly."*

You: "Let me pass you a tissue. Mrs Brown, a small amount of alcohol consumption early in pregnancy has not been linked to an increased risk of developing PPH. Is there anyone you would like me to call to be with you whilst we have this discussion, like your partner?"

Patient: *"My partner has just left to get some supplies."*

You: "Would it help if I spoke to you again with your partner present?"

Patient: *"Yes that would help me."*

You: "We could arrange for me to discuss this with both of you later this evening, if you would like?"

Patient: *"I would really like that."*

What would you ask next?

You: "I know that this is a lot to take in in one go. Would it help if I went through what happened during your caesarean?"

Patient: *"Yes it would."*

You: "As the placenta separates from the uterus and is delivered it is normal for all women to lose some blood. Usually a woman's body has adapted during pregnancy to deal with this blood loss. We also know that women having a caesarean section tend to bleed a bit more than women giving birth vaginally. Unfortunately, some women bleed more than expected after birth, which can lead to a large PPH, which is what we call blood loss within the first 24 hours of giving birth."

Patient: *"But what caused me to bleed so much?"*

You: "There can be a number of causes of excess blood loss, and these may be related to the uterus or the placenta. Looking at your operation notes, the cause of your PPH was secondary to the placenta being low, and I understand that this was the reason you had an elective caesarean section. In your case the placenta was very low, covering the cervix, which we had suspected, and this is called a placenta praevia.."

Patient: *"I see, I think talking to the surgeon that operated on me would help me."*

You: "Is there anything else that is concerning you or anything else I can do to help?"

> 66 **Patient:** *"No, I think I was angry initially because I thought that I lost so much blood because of something I'd done or the surgeon had done."*

You: "Do you feel you have a better understanding of the situation now?"

> 66 **Patient:** *"Yes"*

How would you close the consultation?

You: "I understand why you were feeling angry and I apologise again that you lost a large volume of blood. I will ask a senior doctor to come and speak to you about what has happened. If you write down any new concerns or questions then we can answer those for you. We are going to look after you and ensure you have recovered properly from this. I know you are feeling drained and in pain, so we will give you some strong painkillers and we shall also check your Hb level, which is a blood test. Do you now understand why you developed a PPH now?"

> 66 **Patient:** *"Yes, I can see it was because of a problem with my placenta."*

You: "OK, is there anything else you would like to ask me Mrs Brown?"

The patient has some further questions for you

> 66 **Patient:** *"Is it really rare to have a placenta previa?"*

You: "The incidence is about 1 in every 250 pregnancies."

> 66 **Patient**: *"Why does having a placenta previa increase my risk of PPH?"*

You: "Usually, after the baby is delivered, we will deliver the placenta and we give the mother medication to help contract the uterus. We give this medication to help stop excessive bleeding from the area of the uterus where the placenta was attached. In women who have a placenta previa the medication is not as effective in stopping blood loss, because the placenta is attached to the lower part of the uterus, which doesn't contract as strongly as the upper part. The ineffective contractions generated are unable to stop the bleeding, which can lead to a large PPH. Does that make sense Mrs Brown?"

> 66 **Patient:** *"Sort of, but are certain women more likely to have a placenta previa?"*

You: "We know that women are more likely to develop a placenta previa if they have any of these risk factors [insert risk factors: they have had a placenta previa in a previous pregnancy; they have had 1 or more caesarean sections before; any type of previous uterine surgery; twin or higher pregnancies; multi-

COMMUNICATION

party; older age; cigarette or cocaine use."

SUMMARY

"I know you are angry and I want to reiterate this is not your fault in anyway. I can only apologise that you developed a PPH as a complication of having a low-lying placenta. We shall do everything we can to help you understand what has happened to you. I will ask my senior to come and talk to you about what has happened later today. We are here to answer all your questions and we shall look after you."

 Actor Brief

You are a 44-year-old female teacher, called Mrs Brown who was admitted this morning for an elective caesarean section for a known placenta previa. Unfortunately you developed a large PPH as a compli-cation. You are now feeling really tired and are complaining of being in a lot of pain. You have asked the midwife if you can speak to the on call doctor as you are feeling awful post op. You weren't initially aware that you had a large PPH, and when the doctor tells you, you become really angry because you think it has been caused by something you or the surgeon have done.

Special Instructions: Actor must be angry and confused, especially when talking about her worries regarding why she has developed the PPH and laying blame.

TOP TIPS

✚ When dealing with a patient who is angry because of a post-op-erative complication/medical error, I think as part of your descala-tion techniques, it is vital to apologise, regardless of whether you yourself are personally accountable for the complication/error.

✚ If a patient asks you questions about something you are not confident about, ie. Placenta previa in this case, do not attempt to make things up, as the actors will then challenge you. It is better to be honest and say that you do not know something and then offer them a leaflet and/or for your senior to talk to them.

COMMUNICATION

4.7 | Refusal of Treatment

Scenario

A 26-year-old lady presents with urinary retention. She is 12 weeks into her first pregnancy. Transabdominal and vaginal ultrasound shows a retroverted uterus with a gestational sac and fetus located in the pelvic cavity. A bladder scan shows a 900ml residual volume. She is in significant discomfort but has refused a catheter. You are the SHO on call and have been called to speak to this patient.

How would you begin?

You: "Hello Mrs Darlington, my name is Dr X and I am one of the junior doctors on the gynaecology team. I understand you would like to speak to me about your management. How can I help you?"

❝❝ Patient : *"Yes, I want to speak to a doctor. The nurse wants to insert a tube into me down below, which I will not allow."*

How will you respond?

You: "OK. Would it be helpful if I explained what was going on and the reason behind inserting a catheter?"

❝❝ Patient: *"Yes, because so far I have been scanned and prodded but this pain has not gone away and paracetamol is not working." (appear irritated)*

You: "I can understand the discomfort you must be in. The reason for the discomfort is because you are in urinary retention. That is to say, your bladder is unable to empty as per normal. The reason for this is because your uterus is 'tilted on it'. We call this a retroverted uterus. This causes compression of the opening to the bladder and stops you from passing urine. Does that make sense so far?" (proceeds to draw a diagram)

❝❝ Patient : *"Kind of. So my uterus is squashing my bladder which means I can't pass urine."*

You: "Exactly. Not being able to pass urine is a medical emergency. Your bladder will continue to fill and the discomfort you are experiencing is down to a very full bladder. This is why the paracetamol has not helped."

❝❝ Patient: *"I am in agony. I just want this to be over!"*

You: "There is a solution to this. The plastic tube that the nurses want to insert into your urethra is called a catheter. This will allow urine to pass from within

COMMUNICATION

your bladder into a bag. This will instantly relieve your symptoms. I am very sure of that."

66 **Patient:** *"Is it going to hurt?"*

You: "The insertion of the catheter may be a little uncomfortable. However we do use numbing gel before inserting the soft plastic tubing. As well as the anaesthetic effect, the gel also acts as a lubricant which will ease the discomfort."

66 **Patient:** *"So how exactly do they put the tube in?"*

You: "The insertion of the catheter is done in a sterile way. The catheter is a thin, flexible, soft plastic tube with holes at the end. This plastic tube is connected to a plastic bag. The nurse will insert some numbing gel into your urethra and then insert the thin tubing. Once she sees urine, which confirms the position in the bladder, she will inflate a small balloon with some saline. This small balloon sits at the exit of the bladder and stops it from falling out. It is a quick procedure and the relief will be almost instant." (draws a diagram).

66 **Patient:** *"Hmm. I'm not sure."*

You: "What are your main concerns?"

66 **Patient:** *"Why has this happened to me? Is the tube going to be there forever? Will it harm my baby?"*

You: "Those are all valid concerns and I will aim to address them. This is a rare situation. Urinary retention in a retroverted uterus happens in approximately 1 in 3000 pregnancies. This is because typically as the uterus enlarges, it tilts forwards and expands out of the pelvis. In your situation, it has become wedged in the pelvis. The bladder sits in close proximity and therefore has been compressed leading to obstruction to the flow of urine. Your bladder is currently holding close to a litre. This is the reason for your pain."

66 **Patient:** *"Oh my goodness, a litre!! Right...how long will I have the tube in?"*

You: "I will confirm the duration with my consultant. It may be that we let you go home with a catheter for a week, to allow the bladder to rest."

66 **Patient:** *"A week?! So I have this tube hanging down me for a week?!"*

You: "The catheter can be attached to a smaller, discreet leg bag. You will be aware of it however the benefit of having a catheter is the prevention of urinary retention. After a week, you will return here to have the catheter removed. In this time, the uterus will correct its position spontaneously. Once this has happened, the situation is unlikely to recur."

66 **Patient:** *"Oh ok. So it isn't permanent? What about the baby?"*

You: "No. It is a temporary measure to ensure you do not go into urinary retention again. The baby remains untouched and will not be affected by the catheter. This plastic tube is being inserted directly into your bladder, in a separate compartment to the fetus."

66 **Patient:** *"Oh right. That makes me feel better."*

You: "I'm glad I could be of help and to reassure you. Is there anything else I can help you with?"

66 **Patient:** *"No, that has put my mind at ease. Am I going to have the catheter now?"*

You: "Yes, I will ask one of the nurses to come and insert it in. I will come and review you later and expect that you will feel much better."

How would you close the consultation?

You: "Either myself or a member of my team will come by later to see how you are doing and a consultant will see you tomorrow during the ward round. If you have any further questions, write them down or if they are more pressing, the nurses will know where to find me. I hope that is ok and you are feeling more reassured."

66 **Patient:** *"Yes thank you for your time."*

The patient has a final question

66 **Patient:** *"What are the complications of urinary retention?"*

You: "Complications of urinary retention can include urinary tract infections or damage to the bladder or kidneys"

SUMMARY

"I hope that you are now happy with the plan of a catheter. It is a necessary process and will ease the pain that you are currently in. The reason you went into retention is because your uterus is tilted backwards and compressing your bladder, this typically resolves spontaneously and you will require no further intervention."

COMMUNICATION

Actor Brief

You are a 26-year-old female who is 12 weeks into your first pregnancy. Over the last day, you have been unable to pass urine and is not in significant discomfort. You are worried about the wellbeing of your baby. You are anxious and angry that nothing has been explained to you and that pain relief is ineffective. You have just been told that you will need a catheter and refuse it. This is because you are unaware of its benefits and have concerns surrounding its effect on the baby.

TOP TIPS

➕ Allow the patient to speak and identify the cause for the refusal of insertion. Understanding the patient's ideas, concerns and expectations is key to persuading her to have the most appropriate treatment.

➕ Address her concerns in a sensitive manner using empathy and building rapport

➕ Try to avoid medical jargon when asked about specifics, diagrams and analogies are good at aiding patient understanding

COMMUNICATION

4.8 | Struggling Colleague

Scenario

You are one of the O&G registrars and Emily, one of the F1s, has asked if she can speak to you about something in private. You have worked with Emily for the last 6 weeks and you notice that she seems low in mood and withdrawn recently. You have moved into one of the offices after you have handed a colleague your bleep. Please talk to Emily and answer any questions she may have.

How would you begin?

You: "Hi Emily, good to see how. How can I help you today?"

66 **F1**: *"[Bursts into tears] I just don't think I can carry on doing this job anymore, it is getting far too much for me."*

Continue to gather information, let the patient speak & be sympathetic.

You: "Can I get you a tissue? What is bothering you at the moment?"

66 **F1**: *"I'm just finding it really difficult at work to stay focussed and motivated. I'm feeling quite low most of the time, as I feel like everyone else is just getting on with it and doing really well. I don't feel like part of the team and I'm staying late most nights just so I can finish what I need to."*

You: "I'm really sad to hear that, Emily, as I feel that you are a very good member of the team. Can you tell me if there is anything else bothering you or if there is anything else that has triggered this?"

66 **F1**: *"Just over the past couple of weeks, I've felt very "out of the loop" and not part of the team. I think I'm a bit useless, and I don't know who to talk to. I'm worried that I am letting other people down and that the rest of the team thinks that I am rubbish at my job."*

What will you ask next?

You: "Well I can reassure you that that is not the opinion of other team members. You are always very reliable and do jobs very well. Is there someone or an event that has made you feel like this?"

66 **F1**: *[Again, bursts into tears] "There is one team member in particular who won't stop picking fights with me. He laughs at me when I do anything wrong at all, for example I was unsuccessful at a grey cannula earlier on today and he shouted at me when I asked him if he could*

COMMUNICATION

try. He told me last week that I give a rubbish handover and he thinks I should "take some time to look at my career options." I don't know how much more I can take."

You: "I can see that this is a horrible situation for you to be in, and I can see why you are upset. Let me get you another tissue."

What further questions would you ask?

You: "Is this colleague a senior or is he another F1?"

66 **F1:** *"He is the same level as me."*

You: "Is there anything that may have started this off?"

66 **F1:** *"He's wanted to do O&G since medical school, and he hates it that I really like it too. I don't know if he sees me as competition, but it is becoming unbearable."*

You: "I think the first thing to say is that from my perspective, you are an excellent F1 and I am pleased you are interested in a career in O&G! A key thing here is to discuss these matters with your designated clinical supervisor, as they will be overseeing the team as a whole. I would recommend that you send them an email today to arrange a time to meet up to discuss this with them. It is important to remember that you are of course an important member of the team, and try not to let these events stop you from doing a good job."

66 **F1:** *"I understand, I hadn't thought of seeing my clinical supervisor, thank you."*

You: "You are welcome. I think it's important to do this to make sure you get the senior support and help you need. It may be that your F1 colleague also needs some help as he may be experiencing some difficulties, and finds that letting off steam to you is the way he is coping. Perhaps you could sit down with him just after handover and find out if there is anything bothering him, or if there is anything particular you have done to upset him."

66 **F1:** *"I have been avoiding talking to him, which I think has made it worse because now it is very awkward. I think I will try to talk to him as well, that's a good idea."*

You: "It may be that he needs to talk to his clinical supervisor too. Its important to try and maintain a good working relationship with him, as poor communication might compromise patients'

66 **F1**: *"I know, and that hasn't happened you are right. Thank you very much for the advice and the reassurance."*

How would you close the consultation?

You: "You are welcome. Remember you are very good at your job, have a good chat with your supervisor. I will also always be here if you need someone to talk to, and if you want to I can feed back to your supervisor. In addition to you clinical supervisor, I would also talk to your educational supervisor, if they are someone different, about this. It might also be useful to reflect on this in your e-portfolio. The fact you have come to speak to me about this today is a good thing and reassuring. It is important to not let this affect your work. Your clinical supervisor will be able to help you further."

Emily has one further question

F1: *"Thank you so much for your help and reassurance. It has made me feel loads better. Would you able to talk to the other F1 involved?"*

You: "I think at this point, I wouldn't be able to talk to him directly as I haven't witnessed anything myself. I think the key now is to talk to your own supervisor, and ask for their guidance. If I were to see anything inappropriate during one of my shifts with you both, then I will be able to take some action and report this myself. "

F1: *"OK, thank you."*

SUMMARY

"I hope I've been able to help you today, Emily. It's important to remember that if you feel you are being bullied in the workplace, to any extent, it is important to go to your line manager/clinical supervisor and talk through your options. Other senior colleagues, such as myself, are here and available for you to talk to at any time if you need us. As a team member, you are excellent, and we have no concerns."

 Actor brief

Emily is an F1 on O&G. This is her second rotation, and she is usually very good at her job. She wants to talk to a senior about feeling "rubbish at her job" but deep down it's because she is feeling bullied by another F1, who may be jealous/feels threatened by the fact that Emily also wants to apply for a career in O&G too. She is reluctant to admit that she is being bullied but is receptive to the idea of going to her clinical supervisor for support. She seeks reassurance about her job performance and is really grateful for any positive feedback.

COMMUNICATION

TOP TIPS

➕ Don't be overwhelmed by a colleague showing emotion. Rather treat the matter sensitively.

➕ Don't be quick to take on the responsibility to sort this issue out alone. It is important that the colleague in question is able to talk to their clinical/educational supervisor and gain appropriate advice from them.

4.9 Breaking Bad News (2)

Scenario

Your next patient in clinic, Mrs Smith, is returning after having a CT scan to investigate abdominal bloating and distension. Unfortunately, the CT scan shows an ovarian cancer with ascities. Please let Mrs Smith know the news and answer any questions she may have.

How would you begin?

You: "Hello Mrs Smith, my name is Dr X, I am one of the obstetric and gynaecology doctors. How are you today?"

❝❝ **Patient:** *"I am fine doctor, thank you for asking. I am very anxious about today."*

What would you ask next?'

You: "Ok, Mrs Smith, could you tell me what has been going on so far?"

❝❝ **Patient:** *"Well I noticed a few months ago that I had lost my appetite but my tummy was really swollen and my bowel habit changed- had to run to the toilet! I went to see my GP who did a blood test and referred me in for a scan because he was worried it could be a problem with my ovary."*

You: "Do you know what we problem we were most concerned about?"

❝❝ **Patient:** *"Yes, in case it was a cancer."*

You: "For this conversation Mrs Smith, would you prefer if a family member or friend is present?"

> **Patient:** *"No, I would prefer to find out myself today then tell my children in my own time."*

You: "I do have the result here today, would you like all the information at once or would you prefer some news today and the rest at subsequent appointments?"

> **Patient:** *"I think I would prefer it all today, get it out of the way."*

You: " Well, as you know, we did the CT scan, and unfortunately, I do not have good news for you today. The results are not as we hoped. I am very sorry to tell you that it looks like a cancer of the ovary."

> **Patient:** *[cries] "Oh no…"*

What will you do next?

You: "I am so sorry Mrs Smith, here is a tissue. Would you like a few minutes?"

> **Patient:** *"No, I am ok Doctor. It is just such a shock doctor, even though I thought I was prepared for the worse, I did not think it would happen to me. What does it mean? How do you know it is cancer?"*

You: "I completely understand. I will explain the diagnosis now but if at any stage, you do not understand something or you would like to ask a question, feel free to interrupt me."

> **Patient:** *"Ok"*

You: "The appearance of the mass in the ovary with the raised tumour markers in the blood is why we think it is a cancer. From what it looks on the scan, the cancer is in one ovary and it has grown, or spread, into another tissue in the pelvis."

> **Patient:** *"Oh no, it has spread-what does that mean?"*

You: "from the CT it looks like some of the tumour might have spread just outside of the ovary. When we deal with cancer, it is very important to stage it correctly so we know how to treat it effectively. The CT scan does not tell us everything, we will need to do further investigations to correctly stage it."

> **Patient:** *"I just cannot believe it. I have cancer. So what happens now?"*

You: "To make sure you get the right treatment, we need to complete some more tests. Firstly, we need to do a MRI of your abdomen and pelvis so that we can better image all the structures there. Additionally, we will do a chest x-ray to check that there is no spread to the lungs as ovarian cancer can spread there. Are you ok or would you like a break?"

66 **Patient:** *"I am ok, doctor, thanks for asking. Will I need surgery?"*

You: "Yes, the only way for us to truly know what type of cancer we are dealing with is to take a biopsy of the tissue. We usually carry out a 'debulking' surgery at the same time so that while we can diagnose the cancer, we can also remove the majority of it. Surgery can involve removal of the uterus, both ovaries and fallopian tubes. We also take a sample of abdominal fluid to see if there are any cancerous cells in it. This can be keyhole surgery, laparoscopy, or open surgery, laparotomy."

66 **Patient:** *"I have never even broken a bone, never mind have surgery. This is so much to take in. What do you mean by staging?"*

You: "Staging is basically how we describe how far the cancer had spread. Basically, there are 4 stages, but there are subcategories within each group. Stage 1 means that the cancer is only in the ovaries, stage 2 means that it is growing outside the ovaries but it confined to the pelvis. For example, in your case, from the CT scan, we would deem your cancer as stage 2B as it is confined to the pelvis but had spread past the ovary. Stage 3 is when it has spread outside of the pelvis and into the abdominal cavity or into the lymph nodes. Stage 4 means it has spread to other body organs, such as the liver or lungs."

66 **Patient:** *"Will I need anything else apart from surgery?"*

You: "Surgery is the mainstay of treatment, debulking the tumour and removing any suspicious lesions significantly improves survival. Furthermore, the majority of patients receive chemotherapy as well. Chemotherapy can either be given through the veins or directly into the abdomen. Throughout chemotherapy, response is monitored by CA-125. Radiotherapy is sometimes used in very early tumours as it has not been shown to improve survival in advanced cancers."

The patient has a few questions for you

66 **Patient:** *"Is there anything that increases the risk?"*

You: "It is believed that the more than you ovulate, the higher risk of you are of developing ovarian cancer. This is due to the increased continuous damages to the epithelium on ovulation and the increased risk of mutations when the epithelium repairs and regenerates. Therefore, anything that causes a woman to ovulate would be considered to increase the risk:
- Not having children
- Having children older
- Having your period at a younger age
- Reaching menopause at an older age
- Using HRT for more than 5 years
- Using fertility drugs

Furthermore, being overweight, having a positive family history for ovarian cancer or carrying a 'cancer' gene such as BRCA-1 OR BRCA-2 also have been linked to higher risks of ovarian cancer."

Patient: *"But I had 3 children, doctor, and I never used any fertility drugs. The only thing I ever used was the pill for goodness's sake!"*

You: "Using the pill is actually a protective factor against ovarian cancer, as is breastfeeding and having children. Unfortunately, these things never really make sense."

Patient: *"Chemotherapy as well. I would never have imagined. Is there anything I have done to cause this?"*

You: "Of course not, Mrs Smith. You must not blame yourself; there is nothing you have done to cause this. Is there anything else you would like to ask me?"

The patient has a few more questions for you

Patient: *"Doctor, tell me honestly- am I dying?"*

You: "Mrs Smith, I wish I could answer that question honestly but with the right treatment, there is every chance that you will beat this cancer and be here in 5, 10 years' time. Your prognosis depends on the exact stage of your cancer but for stage 2 cancer, research suggests 55% of women are here in 5 years' time."

Patient: *"Only a half of people, that's so devastating. I do not know anyone who has had ovarian cancer. Is it common?"*

You: "Ovarian cancer is the 5th most common cancer is woman, with over 7,000 people diagnosed each year in the UK."

Patient: *"Is my daughter at an increased risk?"*

You: "Not necessarily, it depends on your family history of cancer. If she would like to be tested, we can offer genetic screening but for the moment, let's focus on getting you better."

Patient: *"I have never heard of anyone in my family having cancer. Hopefully, she will be ok then. I do not even know what the ovaries do! What are they for?"*

You: "The ovaries are a pair of small oval shaped organs in the pelvis, they are the female version of testes. At birth, they contain between 1-2 million ova, or eggs, only 300-400 of these ever mature to be released during menstruation and also secrete the female sex hormones, oestrogen and progesterone."

COMMUNICATION

SUMMARY

"This is horrible news to be given and it can sometimes only sink in when you get home or considering telling your family or friends. If you find it too difficult to tell them and would prefer for me to do it, that is completely fine and we can organise that. . I will arrange an appointment with one of our oncology nurses so that if you or your family have any more questions, there is an opportunity for you to ask them. Also, here are some leaflets on ovarian cancer and what happens from here. We will organise the other scans and I will see you in clinic to discuss the results."

 Actor brief

You are a 68 year old divorced woman with 3 older children and 6 grandchildren. Over the last 2 months you have noticed your stomach is swollen and you have had more diarrhoea. You have hoped that this is just getting older. Upon hearing the news, you start to cry and need a few minute before you can talk. As the scenario progresses, whilst still upset, you are more shocked and focused on the next steps. You are concerned about your daughter potentially getting the disease.

TOP TIPS

➕ Follow the SPIKES format for breaking bad news, ensure you give a warning shot and wait for the patient to ask the questions.

➕ Be empathic and comforting. Place a hand on the patients arm/shoulder if they are upset, or offer a tissue.

➕ Make sure the patient realises that you will see them again and that there are numerous support groups available.

COMMUNICATION

4.10 Self-Discharge (1)

Scenario

You are the SHO on call for the night shift. The nurse on the gynaecology ward has asked you to speak to Mrs Begum, as she is becoming 'distressed'. You are aware that Mrs Begum was admitted yesterday and has been scheduled for laparoscopic surgery to treat a tubo-ovarian abscess in the morning.

How would you begin?

You: "Hello Mrs Begum, my name is Dr X and I am one of the doctors on the obstetrics and gynaecology team who are looking after you. I have come to see how you are and if you had any questions you wanted to ask before your procedure?"

66 Patient: *[teary eyed] "I want to go home now; I have had enough of waiting here all day. No one is doing anything for me."*

Continue to gather information, let the patient speak and be sympathetic.

You: "I am really sorry you are feeling like this Mrs Begum. I understand that you are waiting for surgery tomorrow morning for removal of an abscess. Would it help if I explained to you about what is going on?"

66 Patient: *[sniffling] "Maybe…"*

You: "Can you tell me what you have been told so far?"

66 Patient: *"They haven't bothered to tell me much. Except that I have some sort of an abscess and they think I need surgery for it. I don't know why I have to be operated on, why can't I just go home and complete the course of antibiotics they've given me?"*

You: "I can understand being in hospital isn't pleasant and that most people would much prefer to be at home. You are right though that you have an abscess, which we need to treat so that you feel better. Why do you think that we had advised surgery for treating the abscess?"

66 Patient: *"I don't know, something to do with me having an infection between by tubes and ovaries. My friend had something similar and she only needed antibiotics."*

You: "That's right, you have a tubo-ovarian abscess which is essentially a pocket of pus that forms because of an infection in the fallopian tube and ovary. (draw a picture) If we don't treat the infection, the abscess will grow and may eventually burst, which can unfortunately lead to a life-threatening infection in your abdomen."

66 **Patient:** *"I understand that, but why can't I just go home with antibiotics? Antibiotics are used for infections aren't they? So why would you make someone have surgery if they can be treated with antibiotics?"*

You: "I know this is a frustrating situation Mrs Begum, and you are right in that antibiotics do work against infection. But how successful they are depends on a number of factors, including the size of the abscess. Your ultrasound scan showed that the abscess is a bit bigger than we initially thought it was and you have been receiving antibiotics for almost 48 hours now, but your blood tests and temperature show that the infection is not improving. This means the abscess is not responding to the antibiotics in the way we hoped it would and this means that we need to remove the abscess using surgery in order to treat the infection it's causing. There is also a risk that the abscess may burst without treatment. If this were to happen, it could make you very unwell very quickly. I would be much happier if you were to stay here, as it would be much safer for your own health, as we can monitor you for signs of worsening infection and would be able to operate on you quickly if we needed to."

66 **Patient:** *"I guess I understand why the surgery is important, but I still don't like the idea of it."*

What will you ask next?

You: "Could you tell me if there is anything in particular that is making you worried about the surgery and wanting to go home?"

66 **Patient:** *"I know the surgery is important, but I'm really scared of being operated on…"*

You: "I know that that thought of having an operation is scary Mrs Begum, but the gynaecology team who are performing the surgery are very experienced and have performed this operation many times. We know that any surgery is a significant undertaking and may have its own risks, but we wouldn't have decided on it unless we thought that its benefits far outweigh the risks. Is there anything you are specifically worried about regarding the operation?

66 **Patient:** *"Well, I'm a bit worried about being put to sleep…"*

You: "That is again very understandable. I can explain more about the anaesthesia if you'd like. Before the procedure starts, the anaesthetist will give you some medication that will put you to sleep, which means that during the procedure you won't feel any pain. You are not alone, anaesthesia makes many patients a bit anxious; would it be helpful if the anaesthetic team came to speak to you tomorrow morning and hopefully put your mind at ease?"

> 66 **Patient:** *"Well, I guess that could help put my mind at rest."*

You: "I know that one of the main reasons you want to go home is your concerns about being put to sleep during the operation, but I think it is important for you to know that my medical advice is for you to stay in hospital as this is the safest place for you. Is there anything else worrying you or anything you would like to ask me?"

Answer the patient's questions to the best of your ability

> 66 **Patient:** *[anxiously], "Yes... no ones told me anything about what happens next."*

You: "Would it help if I went through what would happen if you were to stay?"

> 66 **Patient:** *"Yes I think it would. I don't like not knowing."*

You: "We would monitor you throughout the night and make sure you are as comfortable as possible, so hopefully you will be able to get some sleep. We will also continue the antibiotic treatment, and if you need more painkillers you can ask the nurse. We would also ask you to not eat and drink anything tonight. In the morning we will take you through to theatres to perform the operation. The procedure shouldn't take too long, and you should be back on the ward by the afternoon. Would you like me to explain what the procedure involves?"

> 66 **Patient:** *[squirms] "I guess I should know what I'm in for... Will they open me up and leave me with a huge, horrible scar?"*

You: "As I mentioned before, the anaesthetist will put you to sleep, and then once you are asleep we will make a small cut and place a small camera through your belly button and we will then need to make 1-2 further small cuts at the bottom end of your tummy. We will then remove the abscess through these small cuts. The cuts will only be 5-10mm in size and the scars they leave behind will hopefully be very small. If you think it well help, you I can ask my registrar or consultant to come and explain the procedure in more detail tomorrow morning. In the meantime, I can give you some leaflets, and if you think of any more questions you can jot them down and we can answer them later on?"

> 66 **Patient:** *"That makes more sense now. I am sorry for wasting your time doctor."*

You: "Mrs Begum, I assure you that haven't wasted my time, I am just glad that you're feeling a bit better about the surgery now. Is there anything else that is worrying you?"

COMMUNICATION

> 66 **Patient:** *"No, I think I was just frightened of not really knowing why I had to have the surgery."*

You: "And are you happy to stay in hospital now?"

> 66 **Patient:** *"Yes, I feel silly now for even thinking of leaving. I think speaking to the team operating on me tomorrow will also help me."*

The patient has one final question

> 66 **Patient:** "I don't want to waste any more of your time doctor, but why did I get this abscess?"

You: "Mrs Begum, you're not wasting my time, I'm happy to answer any of your questions. There are a number of reasons why women develop abscesses, but most commonly they result from upper genital tract infections, which cause pelvic inflammatory disease (PID)."

How would you close the consultation?

You: "I will let the nurses know that you have decided to stay and to continue your antibiotic treatment. I will also ask one of the senior doctors to come and speak to you about the procedure tomorrow, and they will be able to answer any other questions or concerns you may have. I will also ask the anaesthetist to come and speak to you about the anaesthesia specifically. You are in good hands Mrs Begum. Do you understand that we want you to stay because it's best for your health?"

> 66 **Patient:** *[sniffles] "Yes, thank you for putting my mind at rest."*

SUMMARY

"I can see you have several concerns regarding the operation and being put to sleep, but it is important you stay tonight because we don't want you to go home, become very ill and get rushed back to hospital requiring emergency treatment. I will get the surgical and anaesthetic teams to come and talk to you tomorrow morning and they will able to answer any new questions or concerns you have. We are here to look after you Mrs Begum, and I don't want you to feel like you are wasting our time, as we are happy to answer any more questions you have."

COMMUNICATION

Actor Brief

You are a 34-year-old female receptionist, called Mrs Begum you were admitted yesterday with right lower abdominal pain, fevers and PV bleeding. Relevant past medical history includes treatment for chlamydia, but that was more than a year ago. You have been told that you have an abscess, and have been started on IV antibiotics and have had an USS scan during this admission. You are scheduled for laparoscopic removal of the abscess tomorrow morning. You have asked the nurse if you can speak to the on call doctor as you are very anxious, and you want to go self-discharge. You do not understand why you have to stay in another day for surgery; one of your friends had an abscess and they sent her home with antibiotics. You have never had surgery before and are scared of being put under general anaesthetic and of having a horrible big scar after the surgery.

Special Instructions: Actor should put on the persona of a very anxious and emotionally distressed person, especially when talking about her worries regarding the procedure and when confusing PID with cancer.

TOP TIPS

➕ Always listen to the patient, especially when they want to self-discharge; often it is the case that they feel they do not have enough information and make their own assumptions as a result. You need to get to the core issue to help resolve it. In this case, the patient was worried about anaesthesia and the procedure itself, and she just needed some reassurance and an explanation of what it would involve.

➕ If asked to talk about a procedure or something you are not comfortable or skilled to talk about, do not feel forced to talk about it. You should always tell patients the truth; that you are not experienced, but that you can you get someone more experienced to talk to them. They will appreciate your honesty.

➕ Always ask patients if they have any more questions or concerns, as there may be more than one underlying issue.

COMMUNICATION

4.11 Self-Discharge (2)

Scenario

You are the SHO on call for the night shift and you have been asked to speak to Mrs Smith on the gynaecology ward. You know that Mrs Smith has been scheduled for a laparoscopic removal of an ectopic pregnancy the following morning and is considered not suitable for medical management. You have washed your hands and introduced yourself. Please talk to Mrs Smith and create a management plan.

How would you begin?

You: "Hello my name is Dr X and I am one of the team members in obstetrics and gynaecology. I have come to see if I can answer any of your questions, would you like to ask me some?"

❝ **Patient:** *"Yes I want to go home, no one has explained to me what is going on and I have had enough of being here"*

Continue to gather information, let the patient speak and be sympathetic.

You: "I can understand, I can help explain to you about what is going on, can you tell me what you know or have been told so far?"

❝ **Patient:** *"I know that I am pregnant and that its not in the right place, but I don't see why I have to stay here, I could just go home tonight and come back tomorrow for the surgery"*

You: "I can see that it would be much nicer for you to go home and you are right you are pregnant and it is unfortunately in the wrong place Mrs Smith. There are some important reasons however that we would like you to stay with us over night, rather than go home. Perhaps it will help if I go through these with you? "

❝ **Patient:** *"Yes because no one else has bothered"*

You: "Could you tell me what you know already about an ectopic pregnancy? "

❝ **Patient:** *"Just that it means the baby will not grow"*

You: "That's right, it means that the baby is sitting in the small tube that connects to your womb, rather than in your womb itself, and this tube cannot stretch (draw picture if possible). As the baby grows it can put the tube under pressure and there is a risk that the tube will burst. "

66 Patient: *"I see that makes more sense but why cant I just go home and come back tomorrow? I have all these machines beeping everywhere and I cant sleep, its distressing."*

You: "I know that would be nicer for you, however there is a risk that your tube might burst overnight prior to your surgery tomorrow, if this were to happen it can make you very unwell quickly and it could become life threatening. It would be much safer for your own health to stay here, where we can monitor for this, and if were to happen we would be able to operate on you quickly. "

66 Patient: *"How can you tell if it has burst?"*

You: "That is why we check your pulse and your BP, we monitor these very closely overnight, they give us signs if anything is changing inside your tummy."

66 Patient: *"So the only reason is in case my tube bursts?"*

You: "That is one of the reasons, but also we can make you more comfortable overnight here, for example by giving you strong pain killers."

Explore the patient's ideas, concerns and expectations.

You: "Could you tell me if there is anything in particular that is making you want to go home"

66 Patient: *"Well yes, I have a little toddler at home and I miss him so much, he has never been away from me and I just can't bare to think of him wondering where I am"* [Patient starts crying]

You: "Yes that is very hard, I can see that is a very tricky and upsetting position to be in".

66 Patient: [Crying and hysterical] *"I cant leave him, I am his mother, he is going to think I have abandoned him, he has never been alone before"*

You: "Let me pass you a tissue, is there anyway we can help you with this?"

66 Patient: *"I just want to give him a cuddle"*

You: "Would it help if you spoke to him? we could enable this for you"

66 Patient: *"Yes that would help me, I would really like to speak to him"*

You: "We could arrange for you to call him tonight and in the morning if that would help you?"

66 Patient: *"I would really like that, but I would still like to go home"*

COMMUNICATION

What else would you ask the patient?

You: "I know that and I can understand that there are lots of factors pulling you home, however it is really important for you to know that it is not our advice for you to go home as this could cause you to come to serious harm. Is there anything else worrying you that I could try and help you with"

66 **Patient:** *"I just don't know what to expect from here"*

You: "Would it help if I went through what would happen if you were to stay?"

66 **Patient:** *"Yes it would"*

You: "We would monitor you through the night and we would try and make you as comfortable as possible by giving you pain killers if you needed it. Hopefully you will be able to get some sleep too. We would ask you to not eat and drink and then in the morning we would take you to theatre to perform the operation. The procedure itself is relatively quick and you will be feeling better by later in the afternoon. Would you like to know about the operation?"

66 **Patient:** *"Yes"*

You: "It is an operation where you are put gently to sleep, we then use a small camera to look through your belly button and we can remove the pregnancy and tube from there. If it will help you I can ask my registrar who is more senior to me to come down and talk to you in more detail about this, and I can give you some leaflets."

66 **Patient:** *"I think that would help me"*

You: "I will ask them, is there anything else that is concerning you?"

66 **Patient:** *"No I think I was just frightened of everything, I didn't know what was happening to me and I miss my son. I will stay if I can call my son and know a little bit more about what the procedure is tomorrow."*

How would you close the consultation?

You: "I will talk to the nurses and let them know that you would like to call and speak with your son tonight and in the morning and I will ask a senior doctor to come and speak to you about the procedure itself. If you write down any new concerns then we can answer these for you. We are going to look after you. Do you feel you understand the reason that we want you to stay?"

66 **Patient:** *"Yes, thank you I can see that my tube is at risk of bursting."*

The patient has a few specific questions for you

Patient: *"Is it really rare to get an ectopic pregnancy?"*

You: "The incidence is about 1 in 90, you are not alone."

Patient: *"What about my future pregnancies after this? Will they be affected?"*

You: "For most women an ectopic pregnancy occurs as a one off event and does not happen again. The chance of having a successful pregnancy in the future is good. Even if you have only one fallopian tube your chance of conceiving is only slightly reduced. The chance of having an ectopic pregnancy next time is 7-10 in 100. In your next pregnancy it is advisable to have an USS between 6-8 weeks to confirm that the pregnancy is developing in the womb."

Patient: *"I am sure my friend had an ectopic pregnancy and didn't have surgery? Why do I have to have surgery?"*

You: "The way that an ectopic pregnancy is managed depends on each individual and their personal situation. Some ectopic pregnancies can be managed without any treatment or with a medication called methotrexate. However for this to be safe there are certain requirements, for example a patient needs to have minimal symptoms and their pregnancy hormone level needs to be below a certain level. Unfortunately these options were not suitable for you and would be considered unsafe, potentially putting you at harm."

SUMMARY

"This is not your fault and I can see you are in a very difficult position. It is important you stay tonight because you could become very ill at home and require emergency life saving treatment but I can see that you miss your son dreadfully and you have felt that you didn't know what was going on. We shall do everything we can to help you stay in contact with your son and we shall aim to get you home safely after the procedure. I will ask my senior to come and talk to you about the procedure tomorrow. We are here to answer all your questions and we shall look after you."

COMMUNICATION

Actor Brief

You are Mrs Smith a 32-year-old lawyer. You have been told that you have an ectopic pregnancy that requires removal via keyhole surgery. You are a single parent and have a 3-year-old at home who you have never been away from.

You are very worried about leaving him and are scared that if anything happen to you he will be left without a mother and father.

You don't know very much about the operation and are very anxious.

TOP TIPS

➕ Listen to the patient, get them to talk. There is often an underlying point that you need to get out of the patient. In this scenario it was that she wanted to see her son. Once you have addressed this you can work out ways to solve the problem.

➕ Don't worry too much about the details of an ectopic pregnancy, this is about communication. If you are asked for facts then that is because the actor is pushing you and you are doing well.

➕ Always empathise with the patient. Offer tissues and draw diagrams. Act as you would in real life.

➕ Remember you are not alone. If there is something you are asked explain that you can ask your senior or get them to come and talk to you.

➕ Always let the patient know you are happy to speak to them again, they can write things down if they spring to mind and give them a leaflet.

➕ Don't panic if things appear to be difficult. The actor has often been given a brief to make it challenging for the candidate and can include when to reveal information or if the actor should cry, shout or get angry.

COMMUNICATION

4.12 Contraception

> ## Scenario
> You are an ST1 in a family planning clinic. Sophie, an 18-year-old girl, comes to see you to ask about starting contraception. You have washed your hands and introduced yourself. Please take a history and suggest a management plan.

How would you begin?

You: "Hello Sophie, my name is Dr X, I am one of the obstetric and gynaecology doctors working in the clinic today. How can I help?"

66 Patient: *"Hi, I'm here as I'd like to start the pill please."*

What will you ask next?

You: "OK Sophie, so you're looking to start contraception? I'm sure we can help you, but there are several options available. Why would you like to start the pill, and what do you know about it?"

66 Patient: *"Well I don't know a lot about it, but my friend takes a pill and it works for her. I've just started a new relationship and I don't want to get pregnant, and we don't like condoms."*

You: "Right, well there are quite a few things that we can talk about today. There are several different types of contraception, from barrier methods such as condoms, to inserted or implanted devices and pills. Everyone is different, and you may prefer one method over another – and some aren't actually appropriate for certain people. Would you like me to go over the options?"

66 Patient: *"Yes please."*

Go through the options

You: "Firstly, other than preventing a pregnancy is there anything else that you are hoping that contraception will do for you? Some people use oral contraception for particularly heavy or painful periods for example."

66 Patient: *"Actually I have quite very painful periods, which can be really annoying so if there's anything that can help that then that would be good. Otherwise I want it purely for contraception, I don't want to have children until I'm at least thirty!"*

You: "Well that's a good place to start. As I said before, there are several options for contraception. The first is the barrier method – including male and female condoms, diaphragms and caps. I know you said that you and your part-

COMMUNICATION

ner dislike condoms, but there are advantages – particularly protecting against sexually transmitted infections."

66 **Patient:** *"We've both been to the GUM clinic and have been checked for STIs, so I'm not worried about that. I just don't think I like the hassle of any of those, thank you. What else is there?"*

You: "As you mentioned before, there are oral contraceptives that you can take. The main types are firstly the combined oral contraceptive pill, known commonly as the pill, and secondly the progestogen-only pill – also known as the mini-pill. The mini-pill contains a hormone called progestogen, and it works by thinning the lining of your womb so that an egg is likely to implant, and by thickening the mucus at the opening of the womb (the cervix) to prevent sperm from entering the womb. The pill also uses progestogen, but is combined with oestrogen and it works mainly by preventing maturation of an egg from your ovary, called ovulation. Because of the use of hormones, they both require taking a pill daily but with slight differences. With the pill you take one tablet daily for three weeks and then have a pill-free week, which will trigger the start of a period. With the mini-pill you take the tablet every day and don't have a day off. The mini-pill requires a stricter time period though, and should be taken within three hours of the same time every day although some allow up to 12 hours. What do you think about taking one of these?"

66 **Patient:** *"I'm not sure I would always remember to take a tablet at the same time each day. Is one of them better for my periods than the other?"*

You: "The pill is better for irregular periods than the mini-pill, as the pill-free break can synchronise your periods a little better. It may not work for everyone, but the coil or Mirena are another option for painful periods. There's also a progestogen injection possible."

66 **Patient:** *"Ooh no, I hate injections. Can you tell me more about the inserted devices please?"*

You: "Of course. They are both small devices that are inserted through the cervix into the womb, and sit inside of the womb. The coil is a plastic and copper device and works by causing a small inflammatory response in the womb that reduces the likelihood of an egg implanting into the womb, and also has some spermicidal effects. The Mirena is a plastic device that contains the same progestogen hormone used in the mini-pill, and therefore thins the lining of the womb and thickens the mucus in the same way. Because these devices sit in the womb, they can last for five years – though they can be removed sooner if required."

66 **Patient:** *"That sounds like a fantastic option to me – I won't have to remember a pill, it lasts five years and might sort out my painful periods. That's the one I want please."*

What else would you ask?

You: "Firstly, is there any possibility that you could be pregnant?"

66 **Patient:** *"No, we've been using condoms until I get something else sorted."*

You: "You said that you have had an STI screen. Is there any possibility you could have an infection at present or have you ever had an infection called pelvic inflammatory disease?"

66 **Patient:** *"No to both."*

You: "Have you ever been told you have any abnormalities with your uterus, such as fibroids or an abnormal shape to your uterus?"

66 **Patient:** *"I haven't been told this, but I've never had any investigations that would have told me so."*

You: "That's fine. Have you ever had cancer – particularly breast cancer, ovarian cancer or cervical cancer?"

66 **Patient:** *"No, thankfully."*

You: "Finally, any history of heart disease, liver problems or anything else you've seen your doctor for in the past?"

66 **Patient:** *"Only asthma, and it's well controlled."*

You: "Super, so you don't have any contraindications to having the Mirena. However, I would want to do some cervical swabs and a pregnancy test to just confirm those if that's OK. Shall I tell you about the advantages and disadvantages?"

66 **Patient:** *"Yes please, are there any side effects?"*

You: "The side effects are related to the hormone used, so it's possible to have mood swings, acne, breast discomfort and reduced libido. These will normally show themselves in the first few months and can get better and go completely. Some people will have irregular periods, but again these usually last upto 6 months and then settle down, in fact some women may have no bleeding at all with the Mirena. Some people have heavier periods, but this can also be a sign of infection or pregnancy so if this happens to you then come back for a quick check. Finally, there is a slight increase in risk of ectopic pregnancy. This is when a fertilised egg implants outside of the uterine cavity, or womb. It usually occurs in the Fallopian tube and the risk is that the pregnancy will grow and burst the tube."

COMMUNICATION

❝ Patient: *"Gosh, is that a high risk?"*

You: "Well in any pregnancy there is about a 1% chance of this happening, and although the Mirena increases this risk it is not huge. I can give you some information on the Mirena, which includes an explanation of what an ectopic pregnancy is and the risks and benefits of the Mirena. Would you like that?"

❝ Patient: *"Yes please, I'd also like to know how you insert it – is it an operation?"*

You: "No, it's a very simple procedure that can be done in clinic or at your GP surgery. We would ask you to book an appointment towards the end of your period and when your swabs are back. We would do a urine pregnancy test on the day, and if this and the swabs are negative then we can insert it at the appointment. It can be a little uncomfortable but is a quick procedure and rarely has complications."

❝ Patient: *"OK, this all sounds fine to me. Can we start to arrange everything to do it then please?"*

How would you close the consultation?

You: "Of course. So we've discussed a number of contraceptive options, and you feel that the Mirena is the best option for you. You have no contraindications, so you would be appropriate to have it inserted towards the end of your next period. We'll take some swabs now, and if these are negative then we'll do a pregnancy test on the day of your appointment. I'll give you some leaflets about the Mirena to take home with you, and if you have any further questions or would like more advice then feel free to book another appointment. Is there anything else you wanted to ask at the moment?"

The patient has a few questions for you

❝ Patient: *"Yes, how effective is the Mirena?"*

You: "It is one of the most effective methods of contraception. Only about 2 in 1000 women become pregnant with the Mirena inserted."

❝ Patient: *"OK, and you mentioned complications when it's put in. How likely are these?"*

You: "The most severe complication is perforation of the uterus – where the coil will go through the wall of the womb, however this is uncommon and only occurs in less than 1 in 1000 fittings. It is usually noted at the time of the fitting and would require a keyhole surgery to fix it."

SUMMARY

"Fantastic, I'm glad. It is a very efficient contraception and seems very appropriate for you. If you do decide that you want to get pregnant then it is just as easy to remove, and there is rarely any delay in return of fertility. The Mirena lasts up to five years, and although I'd encourage concurrent use of condoms to prevent any sexually transmitted infections, on its own the Mirena is about 99% effective for this time. I will find you the leaflets I mentioned, and I will give you a contact number to arrange another appointment for insertion. It was lovely to meet you and I'll see you again soon."

 Actor Brief

You are Sophie, an 18-year-old student. You have recently started a new relationship with Sam, and have started sexual relations in the last few weeks. He dislikes using condoms because they are uncomfortable and 'ruin the mood'. You said that you would look into oral contraception providing you both had an STI screen first, which was reassuringly normal. You have a busy lifestyle at university and don't think you'll remember to take a pill every day, but you don't like injections and Sam doesn't like condoms – you want to know if there are any other options. You would like to leave the clinic today with an effective method for contraception, and want it to be an easy method that you don't have to worry about. You'd like it to be highly effective as you don't plan on having children until you're at least 30.

Significant PMH/DH/SH: Asthma, well-controlled and talking salbutamol PRN for this. Living in student accommodation and working part-time in a bar whilst studying sociology.

Special Instructions: Question anything medical that you don't understand, and ask for it to be explained in a simpler language. You are eager to leave the clinic with something effective today, as you don't want this to become a problem in your new relationship, however you will be understanding if it is will explained to you.

TOP TIPS

➕ There is so much information that can be provided on contraception, so be concise to fit it in.

➕ Be aware that they may be requesting oral contraception for reasons other than contraception, such as menorrhagia.

➕ Investigate contraindications and reasons that one contraception may be preferable to another.

COMMUNICATION

4.13 | Explaining a Diagnosis

> **Scenario**
>
> You are an ST1 in the antenatal clinic and Miss Richards has attended for a routine appointment. She is 18 years old and she is twenty-eight weeks into her first pregnancy. She is concerned because her GP detected a 'bug' in her urine and referred her to you. You have washed your hands and introduced yourself. Please take a history and suggest a management plan.

How would you begin?

You: "Hello, my name is Dr X and I am one of the obstetrics and gynaecology doctors. I understand you have some concerns about your recent test result. Would you like to ask me about it?"

66 **Patient:** *"Yes, I had a urine infection recently and my GP seemed particularly worried that it grew something called GBS. I don't know what it is but it sounds serious if they are worried!"*

What will you ask next? Explore her concerns and what she already knows

You: "I understand your concerns, would you like me to help explain this a bit further? What do you know about GBS already?"

66 **Patient:** *"All I know is that it was detected in my urine sample and can cause my baby to be infected when she's born. Is it something I could have got from my ex-boyfriend?"*

You: "Well, firstly I can reassure you that it isn't sexually transmitted so you couldn't have acquired it from your ex-boyfriend. It is actually present in the vagina and bowel of a number of women without causing symptoms or problems to you. Secondly, you are correct that it can cause infection in new-born babies but not all babies born to mothers with GBS will be affected."

66 **Patient:** *"How do I stop my baby from being infected? Is there anything that will make her more likely to get it?"*

You: "There are some increased risk factors. These are having had GBS in a previous pregnancy, having a baby born before 37 weeks gestation, having a long time between your waters breaking and giving birth, and you having a high temperature during pregnancy. Have you had GBS in a previous pregnancy, and have you noticed any high fevers?"

66 **Patient:** *"I've had a few hot sweats but nothing unusual, and this is my first pregnancy."*

You: "Good, that's reassuring. The other way we can reduce your baby's risk of infection is to treat GBS with antibiotics. Because you have a urine infection, we would like to offer you antibiotics now and then we would also offer you antibiotics during labour."

66 **Patient:** *"That sounds like a lot of antibiotics, I'm not sure about that."*

What else would you ask?

You: "Would it help if I explained a bit more about the treatment?"

66 **Patient:** *"Yes please, I think so."*

You: "At present we would give you a short, oral course of penicillin – unless you are allergic. Have you ever had an allergy to penicillin in the past?"

66 **Patient:** *"Not that I know of."*

You: "Good. So after a short oral course we would also give you antibiotics through the vein whilst you are in labour even if you haven't had any more urinary symptoms. This would mean having your baby in hospital, is that something you've thought of before?"

66 **Patient:** *"Yes, and I feel happier having her in hospital anyway. What would happen after that? Would she need further treatment?"*

You: "From the GBS perspective we would monitor your baby for any signs of infection, but otherwise neither of you would require need further treatment. Do you have any further questions?"

66 **Patient:** *"Not at present."*

You: "How do you feel about it now? Would you be willing to consider antibiotics?"

66 **Patient:** *"I feel reassured that it's treatable, and that you say that the antibiotics wouldn't harm my baby. It sounds like it's a good idea, I think I will take them."*

How would you close the consultation?

You: "OK, I'm glad I've explained it sufficiently to you. Perhaps I can provide you with a leaflet with information about GBS so that if you have any further questions it could help. If it doesn't then write your questions down and bring them to your next appointment. So as discussed, we'll start oral antibiotics for your urine infection now and we'll arrange for you to have a hospital birth. When you are in labour we'll give you antibiotics through the vein to reduce the risk of transferring GBS during labour."

COMMUNICATION

66 **Patient:** *"That all makes sense, thank you."*

The patient has a few questions

66 **Patient:** *"Can I ask, is this infection really rare?"*

You: "Well, about 20% of women in the UK actually carry the infection without symptoms. And only 1 in 2000 babies born in the UK are diagnosed with GBS infection. So it's not uncommon."

66 **Patient:** *"OK, and you said that some babies could die from it. How many with the infection would die?"*

You: "That's a good question. The majority of babies with the infection fully recover, but about 20% will have a lasting disability and sadly about 10% will die from it. That equates to a small number of babies thankfully."

66 **Patient:** *"Good, and hopefully my risk will be reduced with antibiotics."*

You: "Absolutely."

66 **Patient:** *"Can I pass it to my baby though breast milk?"*

You: "No that isn't possible – and we would encourage you to breastfeed your baby to reduce the risk of other infections too. Do you have any further questions?"

66 **Patient:** *"No, thank you. I think that taking the antibiotics sounds like the best course of action."*

SUMMARY

"I can completely understand your concerns, and it can be a lot to take in. However, GBS is a treatable infection and the treatment will not harm your baby. Without antibiotics, the risk of transferring the infection to your baby is high, and the complications can be life threatening. As I'd advised, antibiotics are the best treatment and can reduce the risk of transferring GBS to your baby. I'd also like you to be aware that if you went into labour early, at less than 37 weeks, or had a lengthy time between your waters breaking and going into labour, then you should ensure that your doctor or midwife that you have had GBS during this pregnancy. That way we can aim to reduce the risk to your baby further by inducing labour or by careful observation once she is born. I'll find you a leaflet and I'll write you a prescription. Feel free to contact us again if you have any further questions."

Actor Brief

You are Miss Richards, a single, 18-year-old bartender who is twenty-eight weeks pregnant. It is your first pregnancy and you have been very anxious throughout – every (so far normal) symptom of pregnancy that you've had, you've seen the doctor for and you particularly worry about how it all affects your baby girl.

You visited the GP two days ago with pain when you pass urine and he offered you on a course of antibiotics, which you declined as you were worried it would harm the baby. You said you would try cranberry juice and water in the meantime. He called to say that the test had grown a 'bug' and he'd referred you to the antenatal clinic.

You want to know what is going on, why you have an infection and if you could have got it from your ex-boyfriend. You are worried about any sort of treatment in case it harms the baby, and would like reassurance that it'll pass with conservative management.

Special instructions: You are particularly anxious and initially adamant that you wouldn't consider antibiotics as you are sure they harm the baby and you can get antibiotic resistance.

TOP TIPS

➕ Use non-medical language to explain the risks and complications – don't sugar coat it in medical terminology as the patient may not fully understand.

➕ Understand that some people don't like to take antibiotics, particularly when pregnant. Explore why this is and what they understand about the situation.

➕ Offer alternative material, such as a patient information leaflet, and let them know that they can ask further questions.

➕ Remember to presume capacity until proven otherwise – the patient has the right to turn down treatment, as long as they fully understand the risks and benefits, are able to retain and assess it, and can convey their message back to you. Therefore ensure you give them the full information.

COMMUNICATION

MORE ONLINE

www.oginterview.com

 Access Over 500 More Interview Questions

Head over to the Obstetrics and Gynaecology Interview website for the latest news on this year's interviews together with our online O&G interview questions bank featuring over 500 unique, interactive ST1 interview questions with comprehensive answers.

Created by high scoring, successful trainees the website and question bank can be accessed from your home computer, laptop or mobile device making your preparation as easy and convenient as possible.

COMMUNICATION

Printed in Great Britain
by Amazon

38096041R00116